DISTRICT NURSING

DISTRICT NURSING
The Nurse, the Patients and the Work

MOLLIE F. ANTROBUS SRN, NDNCert,
PWT, DipN(London)
Senior Nurse, District Nursing in Newbury, Berkshire

with a Foreword by AINNA FAWCETT-HENESY BA, SRN,
HVCert, FETC
Nurse Adviser, Society of Primary Health Care Nursing
Royal College of Nursing, London

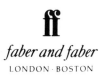

faber and faber
LONDON · BOSTON

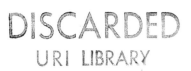

First published in 1985
by Faber and Faber Limited
3 Queen Square, London WC1N 3AU
Printed in Great Britain by
Butler & Tanner Ltd,
Frome and London
All rights reserved

© *M. F. Antrobus 1985*

British Library Cataloguing in Publication Data

Antrobus, Mollie
    District nursing: the nurse, the patients and the work.
    1. Community health nursing—Great Britain
    I. Title
    610.73'43'0941   RT98
    ISBN 0–571–13651–6

Library of Congress Cataloging in Publication Data

Antrobus, Mollie
District nursing.
Bibliography: p.
Includes index.
1. Community health nursing.   2. Home nursing.
I. Title.   [DNLM: 1. Community Health Nursing.
2. Home Care Services.   3. Nursing Process.
WY 115 A636d]
RT98.A57   1985   610.73'43   85–5226
ISBN 0–571–13651–6 (pbk.)

Contents

Foreword

Consumer demand for a genuinely comprehensive health service, the Government's own commitment to primary health care with the emphasis on patients being cared for in their own homes wherever possible, and ever-increasing advances in medical technology have had wide-ranging implications for the district nursing service. Not only have these factors created a phenomenal increase in the work load of the district nurse but, because of the diversity of needs of patients and their families referred to the community services as a result of such developments, the knowledge base of the district nurse has had to expand considerably both in depth and breadth. It is therefore timely that a publication which incorporates so many aspects of the district nurse's new and still developing role should appear on the shelves.

The strength of the book for many will be the strongly practical approach adopted throughout and the way in which it successfully, yet simply, relates theory to practice.

The chapter on the 'Initial Visit' is worth special mention as it sets the scene for the holistic approach to patients and their families evident in all the remaining chapters. It emphasises the importance of the assessment visit and shows how the nursing process actually works in practice; indeed, the chapter demystifies this still widely misunderstood cornerstone of modern nursing practice, and leaves the reader convinced that effective care cannot be assured unless a systematic holistic approach to patient care is adopted and a detailed assessment is carried out on all patients.

The book provides detailed clinical information on a range of medical conditions but again these are treated within a holistic framework; the patient is not 'fragmented' nor the presenting condition viewed in isolation but within the context of the patient's persona as a whole, his immediate family and the wider community.

The book is rich in its application of theory to practice and provides diagrams and illustrations both to simplify the text and to act as quick check-lists on some of the issues raised in the chapters. Comprehensive 'fringe' information on the benefits and services available to at-risk groups is also provided.

The book will be welcomed both as a textbook and a reference work. It should prove to be as valuable to those undergoing district nurse training and new to community care as to those long established in the district nursing service.

> Ainna Fawcett-Henesy BA, SRN, HVCert, FETC
> Nurse Adviser, Society of Primary Health
>   Care Nursing
> Royal College of Nursing, London

Acknowledgements

Thanks are due to many people who have helped in the preparation of this book. Particular mention must be made of the assistance and advice I have received from Catherine Dobson (librarian at the Royal Hampshire County Hospital, Winchester); Wendy Beecher (librarian at the Royal Berkshire Hospital, Reading); Margery Dancer (senior community nurse tutor, Hampshire) and my editor, Miss P. Downie. I would also like to thank Dr Charlotte Kratz who encouraged me to persevere with seeking publication for my manuscript.

I would like to thank the British Diabetic Association, Ames Division of Miles Laboratories Ltd and Surgikos Ltd for providing photographs for inclusion in the book.

Finally, I must thank my husband, Matt, who has put up with much upheaval at home while this book was being written, and who has encouraged me throughout.

M.F.A., 1985

Many changes have taken place in the role, function, education and working conditions of the district nurse during the last 20 years. In spite of this, few books have been written about this type of nursing which is becoming increasingly important as greater emphasis is being placed on community care.

The author became aware of this lack when she herself undertook a course of district nurse training. Later, when she was accompanied on her rounds by student nurses (who have to gain an insight into community nursing as part of their general training), she realised how few books there were about district nursing to recommend as suitable background reading. As a practical work teacher, she found a dearth of books on the practical aspects of district nursing to recommend to nurses undertaking the new mandatory course of district nurse training.

The book describes the clinical nursing and health education aspects of the work of a district nursing sister and was written while the author occupied such a post. The greater proportion deals with the nursing care given to specific groups of patients in their own homes. The shorter section contains information on nursing procedures which may be carried out by the district nurse in the treatment room or patient's home.

Because it is intended as a *practical* account of the district nurse's work, there is little mention of any research on which district nursing practice is based. However, at the end of each chapter, there is a list of further reading. No one book can cover adequately everything which district nurses need to know and they should be encouraged to widen their horizons and read further to extend their knowledge.

When the term 'district nurse' is used, this refers to the district nursing sister, although there are other grades of nurses working in the community such as district enrolled nurses, nursing auxiliaries and practice nurses. There are many male nurses now working in the community and the author apologises to them for using the female pronoun when referring to the district nurse. For simplification, and ease of reading, the patient is referred to as 'he', although with our ageing population and a preponderance of females, in reality the patient is more often a 'she'.

Chapter One

DISTRICT NURSING

'The district nurse is our most widely known, most widely trusted social worker. The rising age of our population, the lack of hospital beds for the old; the discharge of surgical patients from hospital a few days after operation, the growing tendency to nurse children at home and the earlier discharge of patients from mental hospitals are all making her work richer and more diverse and also more exacting' (*Lancet*, 1955). Some 10 years later when the research report *Feeling the Pulse* (Hockey, 1966) was published, a disappointing picture of district nurse isolation was revealed. Over 40 per cent of general practitioners rarely met a district nurse and were ignorant of her qualifications; and district nurses themselves lacked information about the condition and treatment of their patients and complained of poor liaison with health visitors, social workers and hospitals. As many as 30 per cent of district nurses questioned had not even met their local health visitor. Few district nurses at that time had received district nurse training and the majority had little geriatric or paediatric experience.

In the past, district nursing could have been described as a relatively lonely profession. Happily, this is no longer the case. The attachment of district nurses to general practices in 1968, coupled with the reorganisation of the Health Service in 1974 have provided district nurses with unprecedented opportunities for mutual growth and interest. Previous to this the district nurse had traditionally worked on a geographical basis where she had her own 'patch', was well known by the local community, but had little, if any, contact with the many general practitioners whose patients lived in her area. Often the doctor himself did not know all the district nurses who could be caring for his patients and, as a result, misunderstandings easily arose and patients were given conflicting advice.

It was for these reasons that nurses and doctors got together to discuss alternative methods of caring for the health of the community and the idea of a primary health care team and the attachment of district nurses and health visitors to group practices of doctors evolved.

THE PRESENT TIME

Since 1968 group attachment has become the norm, although in some rural areas the district nurses still cover a geographical area because the population is small and more widely dispersed. In these circumstances nurses (known as 'triple workers') are employed: these have a three-fold function and possess district nursing, midwifery and health visiting qualifications. In other areas the district nurse may also carry out domiciliary midwifery duties if the female population of child-bearing age is not too large. The nurse in this case is known as a district nurse/midwife.

The more usual arrangement is for individual district nurses, health visitors and midwives to be attached to a group of general practitioners, who work from a health centre, medical centre or group practice. These nurses care only for patients who are registered with these doctors.

Primary health care services and teams

The primary health care services usually provide the first point of contact between the public and the National Health Service. They aim to:

1. Provide personal care for the public in their own homes.
2. Offer protection against illness and infection.
3. Give continuing support to patients and families throughout illness and rehabilitation or the terminal phases of disease.

Primary health care provides care for patients with varying diseases, both physical and mental, as well as attempting to alleviate any social factors which may affect the patient's recovery. A team can only function efficiently when each member recognises and respects the talents of the others in the group and is able to judge when these skills can be of value. For a primary health care team to work well there must be agreement on how best the team can meet the specific needs of a particular practice population. Consequently, meetings, discussions and the occasional case conference should be an integral part of the programme of all team members.

There is a gradual trend throughout Europe towards concentration on the maintenance of health rather than simply to respond to disease. The official policy in Britain now is to spend more money on people rather than on buildings, and on the community personal health services rather than on institutional care. The main object of future years will be the development of primary health care teams which can foster prevention in the community, cope with the increasing numbers of elderly and disabled and reduce the demands on the acute hospital services.

Because of the changing needs of the population, the training schemes for the primary health care team members must be adapted accordingly: increasingly more attention is needed in all aspects of prevention. Doctors, nurses and health visitors can advise and help individuals to help themselves because it is the positive attitude and willingness of the individual to help himself which aid prevention and rehabilitation.

THE WORK OF DISTRICT NURSES

At present there are three grades of nursing staff caring for patients in the community. The district nursing team is led by the district nursing sister (district nurse), a registered nurse who has completed a post-basic course in district nursing and possesses a National Certificate in District Nursing (NDN). This training is now mandatory in order to practise as a district nurse and take responsibility for managing a caseload. Working under her direction there may be district state enrolled nurses (who have completed a district nursing course for enrolled nurses) and in some areas nursing auxiliaries are also employed to work in the community.

Provision of nursing care to the sick in their own homes

The district nurse is responsible for making the initial visit to the patient in his home. She will assess the needs of the patient and his family and plan the care that her team of nurses will be able to give; she will also discuss with the family how they can participate in the caring process. She can mobilise any additional help that is needed and allocate duties to her nursing team. She may well decide to participate actively in that care herself. Conversely she may only visit the patient on a weekly basis to evaluate progress and change the nursing care plan if necessary. This initial visit is discussed at length in Chapter 2.

Liaison

The district nurse must discuss any changes in her patient's condition and care with the general practitioner and others involved in providing care. She should keep in contact with the community liaison sisters at the local and district hospitals so as to make quite sure that all patients leaving hospital receive continuing care where necessary. It is also vital that other nursing colleagues looking after her patients when she is off duty are kept up to date with changes in the caring programme.

In fact the district nurse liaises with many people who are involved in the care of her patient, for example

family and carers
physiotherapist and occupational therapists
social workers
chiropodists
day hospital staff
home help and meals on wheels organisers
primary health care team members
outpatient clinic staff
voluntary agencies, clubs and day centres
other nurses both in hospital and in the community

Health centre clinics

The district nurse may be required to take part in the running of a nurse's clinic, generally held in a health centre treatment room. Alternatively, if the demand is great, GPs may employ their own full-time nurse in the health centre to provide nursing care for all patients sufficiently mobile to attend her clinic. This position is unlike that of the district nurse who, because of her need for mobility, can usually only spare one hour of her time each day for the clinic and often has to see patients by appointment only. The Appendix on page 160 describes some of the nursing procedures carried out in the health centre treatment room.

In some areas district nurses may run their own clinics specialising in one specific health or screening problem, for example varicose ulcer clinics; diabetic clinics; well-woman clinics; hypertension screening clinics and screening clinics for elderly patients.

Administration

The district nurse also has an administrative role to play within the nursing team. She must maintain accurate records of each patient's care. A nursing record card is left in the patient's home and details of the care given are noted down by each nurse who visits the patient. Most areas are now using the nursing process as a method of providing nursing care. In this case it is the nursing care plan which the sister leaves in the home.

She is responsible for delegating the nursing caseload to the nurses in her team; she needs to ensure that not only are they capable of carrying out the allocated care proficiently but that they have had adequate training and supervision. All nurses working in the community must record and submit monthly returns to their nursing officer. These include:

1. Details of the number of patients visited, their ages and the kind of nursing care given.
2. Details of travel, mileage and the cost of petrol and car maintenance.
3. Details of telephone calls made to colleagues to pass on information about patients to be visited the next day.
4. Itemised salary claim forms giving any overtime worked or periods of duty when on call.

In addition the district nurse may be required to submit a report on any seminars, conferences or study days which she has attended (and indeed should be encouraged to attend). She may have to write a report about the care given to a specific patient, especially if there has been a complaint. Because the district nurse works very much on her own this is another reason for the emphasis on regular and accurate record keeping and the reporting of any accidents. She must ensure that she and her team implement, where appropriate, district policies and procedures. Each nurse working in the community has the responsibility for managing her own caseload and should consider individual patient need, geographical constraints and the need to liaise with other team members when planning her working day and its priorities.

Teaching responsibilities

Students in the community

In July 1977 the EEC directives on nursing were signed. As a result all student nurses must have clinical experience in seven specialties, including home nursing. However, training in community care cannot be looked at in isolation from a student's overall training programme. Ideally it should be a logical part of that programme and wherever possible follow in continuity. The General Nursing Council (GNC) 1977 *Educational Policy Document* stated that all students must spend a minimum of 60 hours in the community with the district nursing sister and/or health visitor. However there is no compulsion for the pupil nurse to gain community experience, although it is stated that 'any opportunity should be taken to include some aspects of community care, preferably by incorporating suitable placements within a unit of experience'. Thus the district nurse has only a very short period of time in which to instruct the student in all that she needs to know about nursing patients in their own homes. For this reason all aspects of community care must be emphasised throughout the training period, and continuing care discussed, whatever disease process or nursing specialty is under consideration at a particular time.

The district nurse sometimes has the responsibility of taking a primary health care team colleague out with her for the day so that the student can have some insight into the work of the district nurse as a nursing member of the team. Such students might include pupil midwives, student psychiatric nurses, health visitors and social workers or maybe a medical student or GP trainee.

This of course means that extra strain is placed on the community nursing services and often has a consequential effect on patients when different people visit them in their homes with 'their nurse'. For the nurse it means extra time spent in planning and carrying out a teaching programme.

District nursing students are placed with practical work teachers (PWT) for practical experience of district nursing during their six-month training. Practical work teachers are experienced district nurses who have completed a course of training to prepare them for this extra teaching role.

Voluntary agencies

The district nurse is often asked to lecture to various voluntary organisations on subjects related to her work; she may talk to members of the British Red Cross Society or the St John Ambulance Brigade about the principles of home nursing, first aid and home safety and/or be asked to examine the members on these subjects. The individual nurse must decide whether she wishes to participate in this type of teaching as it is not included in her job description and may be on a voluntary basis.

Patients and relatives

Because the district nurse is not able to give 24-hour care to her patients she must show them how to help themselves, and carers must be taught how to nurse the sick person until the district nurse calls again. In the case of a patient who is terminally ill, often all that is needed is basic nursing care to ensure that the patient is both comfortable and contented and to prevent the development of any further complications owing to the patient's weakness or inability to cope with practical bodily needs.

When the patient suffers from a chronic disabling condition, a long-term care and rehabilitation programme is part of the district nurse's teaching.

Health education

Health education is considered an integral part of the work of the district nurse and because she visits people in their own homes she is in an ideal position to advise patients and relatives on such subjects as home safety, diet, hygiene, misuse of drugs, smoking, hypothermia and the need for adequate exercise. These are just a few examples of some of the aspects of health education carried out by the district nurse. Various helpful leaflets are available from the local health education department, as well as voluntary organisations (see p. 191).

Counselling responsibilities

The district nurse meets many patients who have a desperate need for counselling as well as physical nursing care. Listening can sometimes be as therapeutic as actually carrying out nursing or medical procedures. Examples include mastectomy and stoma patients who are concerned about the loss of their body image and who are worried about their future prognosis; the handicapped who feel that they are a burden to their caring families and the dying and bereaved (who are considered in more detail in Chapter 6).

The district nurse has many roles to play in the community. Sometimes she visits a home only to give support and advice to the patient and his family. She may mobilise other agencies more suited to meet her patient's needs. She needs a knowledge of the facilities available locally and whom to contact and when.

The district nurse is a visitor to her patient's home and can be (but rarely is) refused entry. She must be particularly careful when using articles and equipment belonging to her patient. She must not damage his furniture or floor coverings with the lotions or equipment that she uses. She must be economical in her usage of electricity and items obtained on prescription or provided by the health authority. She has legal responsibilities in respect of giving the correct dosage of drugs as ordered by the GP; she has a professional responsibility for her own standards of practice and for ensuring that the equipment used is safe and in working order. She has a responsibility to ensure that the carers are aware of how to care for the patient in her absence and are confident in their handling of any equipment involved. She must report any accidents which occur to the patient, carers or herself and record these in the accident book. Finally, she is responsible for the upkeep of her car within legal stipulations and health authority requirements.

Many district nurses are quite content and receive great satisfaction from the work they do. Others may eventually wish to progress from nursing in the community and there are various opportunities open to them including practical work in teaching, district nurse tutoring, administration, community liaison, health visiting, specialisation and research. Whichever she chooses, the district nurse of today will have benefited immensely from the experience of caring for patients in their home environment.

REFERENCES

General Nursing Council (1977). *Educational Policy 1977.* General Nursing Council, London.

Hockey, L. (1966). *Feeling the Pulse. A Study of District Nursing in Six Areas.* Queen's Institute of District Nursing, London.

BIBLIOGRAPHY

Berber, J. H. and Kratz, C. R. (jt eds) (1980). *Towards Team Care.* Churchill Livingstone, Edinburgh.

Clark, J. and Henderson, J. (jt eds) (1983). *Community Health.* Churchill Livingstone, Edinburgh.

Chapter Two

THE INITIAL VISIT: APPLYING THE NURSING PROCESS

The process of nursing is a theoretical framework which can help the district nurse to plan nursing care for each patient according to his individual needs. When using this process the nurse is moving away from the task-orientated approach to nursing care towards a problem-orientated approach of total individual care. There are four main stages to the nursing process: assessment, planning, implementation and evaluation.

ASSESSMENT (Fig. 2/1)

The first visit by the district nurse is usually an assessment one to identify the actual and potential problems of the patient and his family. It may be that a comprehensive assessment cannot be carried out until the second or third visit, with urgent needs being dealt with initially. Assessment is continuous for the district nurse, who is constantly observing and interacting with her patient. She learns of his problems and fears, his lifestyle, the effect of his illness and his social milieu. It is hoped that the patient learns the nurse is a professional caring person, interested in his problems and hoping to help resolve them.

When a patient and family are worried and tense, reassurance is not merely a question of what the nurse says: the most effective reassurance comes from her nursing and one of the most important things that she can do is listen to her patient. Listening allows him to feel that someone understands, and the district nurse must be a good listener and skilled in interpersonal relationships.

Referrals

Referrals to the district nurse for a visit to a new patient in the community may come from numerous sources including general practitioner, district general hospital (community liaison sister),

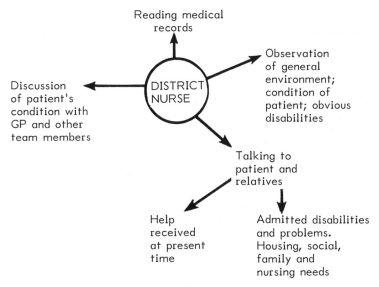

Fig. 2/1 Assessment on the 'first visit'

community hospital, following day-case surgery at a local hospital, health visitor, midwife, community psychiatric nurse, factory doctor or industrial nurse, social worker, home help organiser, geriatric assessment ward or day hospital, rehabilitation unit, physiotherapist or occupational therapist, practice nurse, voluntary agencies, or relatives or friends of a sick person.

Following the initial referral the district nurse should obtain any relevant information about the patient from the primary health care team and other sources such as the patient's medical notes. She should record in her own nursing history any details of his previous medical history which are relevant to her present referral; also to be recorded are recent investigations, therapy and medication.

The actual first visit

Before the nurse even meets the patient she can obtain a general impression of the neighbourhood in which he lives, and as she walks towards it, the upkeep of the house and garden can be noted. Inside the house the nurse observes the patient's personal environment and notes the following: is it tidy or cluttered; is there adequate lighting or a dull, dimly-lit atmosphere; the temperature of the home; the state of cleanliness (décor, peeling wallpaper, rotting wood, condensation, damp patches and other health hazards); and the smell of mildew, urine or faeces.

Introducing herself to the patient and relatives the nurse explains why a visit has been requested. She can then encourage them to tell her about the onset of the present illness. She may ask about the doctor's instructions to them, what medicines the patient is taking and how often, the patient's mode of living before his illness, and his attitude to this illness.

Many district nurses use the activities of daily living method of assessing their patients. This highlights how a disease process has affected their ability to care for themselves and to lead normal, healthy, active lives. The nurse records what the patient can or cannot do for himself. She discovers his normal habits and any deviations from that normal may be recorded as problems. The district nurse is also making observations of her patient during this assessment. While talking to the patient the following observations can be made: is the patient wheelchair bound, confined to an armchair or bedfast; his state of consciousness; are there paralysis, stiff or absent limbs, swollen joints, loss of vision or hearing, aphasia and/or difficulty in communication, dyspnoea, wheezing, a productive or dry cough, cyanosis or oedema?

Activities of daily living assessment

The following is a check-list of factors which the district nurse may wish to consider when considering her patient's ability to cope with the activities of daily living:

Communication

Speech – the presence of dysphasia, aphasia, dyslexia, stuttering. Can the patient read and write? What is his native language and the extent of his vocabulary?

Hearing – the presence of increasing deafness or wax in the auditory canal. Does he wear a hearing aid? Is it functional? Has he got batteries for it?

Vision – the presence of cataract, diabetic retinopathy, eye infections, an artificial eye. Is his eyesight good? Does he visit the optician regularly? Does he wear glasses for distance or reading?

The district nurse may notice during the assessment interview that the patient is communicating in a non-verbal way. His facial expression, posture, fumbling actions, looking away and avoiding eye contact and various gestures are all significant ways of communicating a message to the nurse. The tone of his voice can indicate an emotional state. Listlessness might mean depression and a loud voice could indicate anxiety or deafness. While obtaining the nursing history it is important that the district nurse should use language which is simple and appropriate to the patient's understanding.

Personal cleansing and dressing

Personal hygiene: Is the patient able to wash and bath himself? Can he wash his hair? If the patient is female, does she visit the hairdresser or have a home visit from one? Are there any problems with clothing or the patient's ability to dress himself? What is the condition of his hair and scalp?

Condition of the skin and feet: The district nurse should observe the following while she is bathing her patient: any skin problems such as bruising, oedema, infections, rashes, infestations, dehydration or pressure sores. A Norton Scale rating (see Table 6/1, p. 65) at this stage is useful to identify potential problems and measure progress at a later evaluation. She should also record whether the patient's skin is cold and clammy, dehydrated or flushed. Corns, callosities, thickened toenails and other deformities should be noted. The patient's ability to care for his own feet and the need for the services of a chiropodist are also very relevant.

Oral hygiene: Can the patient care for his own oral hygiene? Has he still got his own teeth and, if so, what is their condition? If he has dentures, does he wear them and what is their condition? Does the patient regularly visit the dentist? What is the condition of his mouth? Does he suffer from mouth ulcers, a sore tongue or halitosis?

Breathing

The district nurse can observe the patient's respiration rate and rhythm during the interview. She should note any cyanosis or dyspnoea on exertion. She should ascertain from the patient whether his breathing is normally like this; whether he smokes and if so, how many? Does he have a chronic cough? Does he expectorate sputum and what colour is it? Is he able to climb stairs? How many pillows does he need at night? Has he always needed this many? Does he need oxygen?

Eating and drinking

The district nurse should ask the patient about his normal dietary habits and his particular likes and dislikes. Any religious or medical restrictions in his dietary intake should be noted. She should ask about his ability to partake of a normal diet, or whether he can only manage a soft or fluid diet. Can he feed himself or does he need assistance? Does he suffer from dysphagia, nausea, vomiting or dyspepsia? Is the patient thin and emaciated or, alternatively, obese? What is his fluid intake throughout the day? Does he take alcohol regularly?

Elimination

Micturition: The patient's normal pattern of micturition should be noted together with any recent deviations. She should record symptoms of polyuria, dysuria, nocturia, pruritis, frequency, urgency or burning on micturition. Is the patient incontinent? Does he have a catheter or a stoma which is draining urine? Does he need special equipment? How far is it to the toilet from the patient's normal base and how suitable are the toilet facilities? (See also Chapter 10.) A specimen of urine should be obtained for urinalysis after the interview if this is possible. If not then the nurse will ask the patient to save a specimen for her to test on her next visit.

Defaecation: What are the patient's normal bowel habits and have these changed recently? Does he suffer from constipation or diarrhoea? Has he a known organic disease? Does he get pain on defaecation? Does he suffer from faecal incontinence or haemorrhoids? Is faecal incontinence a problem? Does he have a stoma? Does he take laxatives?

If the patient complains of rectal bleeding then he will need to be examined by a doctor. The nurse may be asked to obtain a specimen of faeces to be sent to the laboratory. If the problem is one of incontinence then the district nurse should carry out a rectal examination to eliminate the possibility of faecal impaction.

Menstruation: If this is relevant then the district nurse should ask the patient about her normal menstrual cycle and whether the periods are regular, heavy or painful. Other relevant questions include enquiry into whether the patient has had any gynaecological operations; whether she takes a contraceptive pill; whether she has a vaginal discharge. Details of pregnancies should be recorded and any problems noted.

Mobility

This is of particular importance to the patient wishing to remain in his own home. Does he suffer from problems relating to mobility? Does he normally go out of the house? What does he see as the cause of his decreased mobility? What are the factors which limit his independence? Is he chairbound or bedfast? Does he have a wheelchair? Is his house adapted for wheelchair living? Has he any upper or lower limb defects? Are his joints restricted in their movement by pain or stiffness or oedema? Have any therapeutic immobilising procedures been carried out? Is he easily fatigued? What does he know about his own particular need for exercise? Has he got muscle wasting, paralysis, deformities or contractures?

Maintaining a safe environment

Here the district nurse should record her own observations plus any made by the patient or carers. She should note home hazards, fire dangers, and any impairment of the patient's vision, hearing, mobility or memory which are affecting his safety. How aware is the patient of the dangers within his environment? Is there a potential risk of hypothermia, infection or tablet overdosage? How safe is the equipment being used by the nurse and carers? Does the patient suffer from postural hypotension or falls?

Recording any factors in the patient's environment which could be of danger to him is not sufficient. The district nurse must also warn the patient and carers and advise them how to combat these dangers.

Pain and discomfort

Nothing is more tiring and depressing than pain. When patients have pain the district nurse must find out more about the type, for example whether acute or chronic. The completion of a pain chart by the patient may give a clearer picture. The nurse should ask the patient to point to the source of the pain. Is it related to movement or food? How long has he had it? Is he taking analgesia? How effective is the medication? Is he using other remedies to relieve the pain? Is the doctor aware of his pain problem?

Sleeping

Lack of sleep can also be very wearing for the patient. It could be linked to the pain problem, or could be due to worry or depression. The district nurse should find out what time her patient normally goes to bed and how long he usually sleeps before waking up or getting up. Does he take daytime naps? Have there been any recent changes in his sleeping pattern? Does he rely on hypnotics or other remedies to help him get to sleep? Has he got something that is 'playing on his mind'?

Change in body image

This is sometimes a difficult subject to broach, and patients may not wish to talk openly until they have got to know and trust their district nurse. They may be having marital problems with difficulty in establishing normal loving relationships. They may be feeling that they are no longer attractive to their partner because of disfigurement, the loss of a limb or a breast. The creation of a stoma can lead to psychological as well as sexual problems. Other surgical procedures, radiotherapy or chemotherapy can have equally distressing effects. The district nurse must be very tactful and sympathetic in her approach to these patients.

Psychological assessment

Psychological assessment of the patient is something which a district nurse will build up gradually. Obvious problems will be noted at the first visit but other clues tend to slip out as the district nurse and her patient get to know and trust each other more. Factors and observations which should be included in this assessment are:

Orientated or confused
Awareness of diagnosis implications
Level of distress
Patient's/family's wishes
Level of intelligence
Temperament and personality traits
Apprehension/financial or family problems/work security

Mood – anxious, depressed, euphoric, withdrawn or aggressive, friendly, realistic

Beliefs/ambitions/confidence/self-respect/expression of feelings

Psychiatric disorders.

Psychological factors can have an effect on a patient's recovery from physical illness; identifying such problems helps the district nurse in her efforts to give total patient care.

Social assessment

Once the assessment of her patient has been completed the district nurse should discuss and observe his social environment so that a decision can be made as how best to provide for the needs of the patient and his family.

Type of housing – council, rented or privately owned
   – house, bungalow or flat
   – terraced, semi-detached or detached
   – adaptations needed

Type of heating – open fire, gas, electricity or oil

Type of cooking – electricity, Aga, oil or gas (mains or Calor)

Water supply – mains or well
   – availability of hot water

Sanitation – mains sewerage, water closet and cesspit, chemical closet
   – situated indoors or outside

Area – urban or rural

Availability of local services – isolated, on a bus route, near local shops, near doctor's surgery

Ability to cope with domestic activities – shopping, cooking, cleaning, laundry, heating

Help received – professional support (health visitor, social worker, occupational therapist, physiotherapist, GP, speech therapist, chiropodist, Macmillan nurse, community psychiatric nurse)
   – home help (how often?)
   – meals on wheels (how often?)
   – voluntary visitors
   – good neighbours
   – family support (who is involved and what do they do?)

– holidays arranged
– aids provided (type and source of supply?)
– assistance provided by family and friends

Social activities – hobbies, sports or games, clubs, library, outings, day centre, luncheon club, voluntary visiting, church attendance, holidays, bingo, watching television

The nurse must also discover how the patient's present illness has affected his participation in these social activities.

Finance

This is a difficult subject to broach as many people are too proud to admit that they do have financial problems and of course illness makes the problems worse. The nurse should note any obvious signs of poverty plus the fact that the patient needs numerous prescriptions. Relatives may have to take time off from work to care for the invalid and if this is likely to be a long illness then they may well lose their jobs. Other factors include the need for extra heating or a special diet. Also what allowances are received by the patient or his carers? (See p. 188.)

PLANNING CARE (Fig. 2/2)

Having assessed the needs of the patient and family, the district nurse should discuss and agree with them a suitable plan of care. This plan should take into account the nursing and caring needs of the patient and those of the family; the possible need for rehousing or home adaptations; whether household help or help for employment and rehabilitation, companionship and financial assistance are required.

Nursing needs

When planning nursing care the district nurse considers the following probable needs of the patient:

1. The need for general nursing care, which includes assistance with personal hygiene, and bathing, mouth care, care of the skin and pressure areas, help with getting dressed, feeding and prevention of constipation.
2. The need for regular injections, the dosage, method of injection and the frequency.

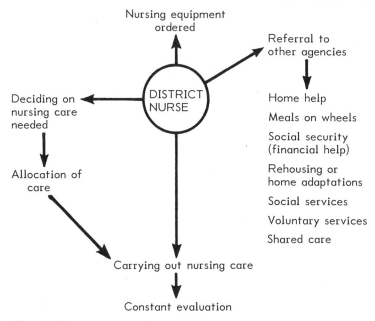

Nursing equipment
ordered

Referral to
other agencies

DISTRICT
NURSE

Deciding on
nursing care
needed

Home help

Meals on wheels

Social security
(financial help)

Allocation of
care

Rehousing or
home adaptations

Social services

Voluntary services

Shared care

Carrying out nursing care

Constant evaluation

Fig. 2/2 Planning care on the 'first visit'

3. The need for the provision of nursing equipment such as commodes, bedpans, urinals, feeding cups, bedcradles, sheepskins, ripple beds, air rings, liquidisers, backrests, wheelchairs and hoists.
4. The need for regular dressing of wounds, ulcers, or pressure sores, and the type of dressing to be used; the frequency with which the dressing is to be carried out and whether a wound swab is required to identify any bacterial infection.
5. The need for rehabilitation and its likely form. If possible the patient should be referred to the physiotherapist or occupational therapist.
6. The need for dietary advice.
7. The need for supervision of medication.
8. The need for assessment, advice and treatment of incontinence and the provision of aids.
9. The need for help and education in the care of a stoma.
10. The need for recatheterisation and advice on catheter care.

11. The need for instillation of eye or ear drops and how often this is to be carried out.
12. The need for adequate rest and sleep.
13. The need to maintain body temperature, and for early recognition of the possibility of hypothermia.
14. The need to avoid further deterioration in the patient's condition caused by home hazards, and consequently the need for health education.
15. The needs of the patient for stimulation, occupation and recreation.
16. The need of the patient to express his fears, opinions, emotions and worries.

The needs of each patient are different and must be considered when planning nursing care. The social situation of each patient also differs and may affect the way in which nursing care can be given.

Family requirements

The nurse should also consider those helping with the care of the patient. Their needs include:

Help with the caring process
Advice on how to care for the patient
Provision of aids and equipment to assist in nursing the patient
Possible financial assistance in the form of Attendance, Invalid Care, Mobility, and other allowances (see p. 188)
Relief from caring in the form of shared-care arrangements and short-stay holidays
Knowledge of the condition of the patient and what to expect in the way of disease manifestations and deterioration
Knowledge of whom to contact (and how) if problems arise.

When caring for a chronically sick person in his own home the actual care given may be less effective because of the unsuitability of the house. The nurse can advise the family on how to apply for rehousing on medical grounds and the general practitioner will have to be asked to complete a form to support this request. Many people do not want to move from their homes, however unsuitable they may be. In such cases the nurse has to be adaptable and practical in her planning of nursing care.

Housing needs

These may include:

(a) The need for ground floor accommodation for a patient who is unable to go up and down stairs, or who is wheelchair bound.
(b) The need for warden-controlled housing for elderly people.
(c) The need for specially adapted accommodation for the disabled to enable them to remain independent.
(d) The need for rehousing because of health hazards from dampness and condensation, dangerous structural defects, lack of sanitary provision and possible infestation by rats, mice or insects.

Alternatively, housing adaptations can be sufficient to allow a patient to remain in his own home. These may include:

(a) The provision of ramps for the patient in a wheelchair.
(b) The installation of a hoist in the bedroom and bathroom.
(c) The fixing of extra banisters or grab rails.
(d) The lowering of working surfaces.
(e) The widening of doorways and the lowering of locks.
(f) The installation of showers and the provision of bath aids, raised lavatory seats, etc.

The district nurse must liaise with the local social services department and housing department for housing/adaptation assessments. Other aspects of planning care to be considered include dealing with the patient who is unable to cope with household chores and shopping. The nurse may contact the home help service, the organiser of the meals on wheels service, the good neighbour scheme organiser, any appropriate voluntary agency and the WRVS.

Many house-bound people require companionship and recreation. All too often the district nurse visits people who are suffering from social isolation in addition to their physical disabilities. While planning nursing care for such a patient, she should consider the possibility of the following solutions to this problem (if the patient so wishes):

Voluntary visiting schemes
Local clubs for the elderly and disabled
The existence of day centres
Adopt-a-granny schemes

Good neighbours
Specific visiting, for example Multiple Sclerosis Society visitors
Holidays
Luncheon clubs
Mobile library services.

Financial needs

The sick patient who is out of work, has a low income or is elderly, may be unaware of the financial assistance which is available. Therefore in her planning of care the nurse should advise the patient on how to apply for the following benefits: supplementary benefits or pensions; help with heating costs; attendance allowance; mobility allowance; invalidity pension; non-contributory invalidity pension; financial assistance from voluntary groups.

Once the problems and needs are identified then the district nurse, together with the patient and carers, can set reasonable goals or objectives around which to plan nursing care. Planning care in order to achieve these goals involves the district nurse in decision making once she has considered available resources (including personnel, support services, carers, the patient's physical environment and suitable equipment) and the possible alternative nursing interventions.

When considering the resources available in the patient's family and how much these should be used in caring for the patient the nurse must assess the following:

(a) General intelligence of the caring family
(b) Age, physical health and strength of family members
(c) Availability of family and friends
(d) The personal relationship between patient and relatives
(e) Resourcefulness of family members, willingness and ability to learn and adapt to a new situation
(f) Financial and social position.

The deciding factor lies in the willingness of the family to participate in caring for a sick relative. Only then can the nurse think of how and in what form this participation in patient care should take place. If the family support is inadequate and the patient's needs are not being met then progress will be slow and other avenues of help may need to be explored.

A nursing care plan is then completed which should state all the nursing activities to be carried out, how often and by whom. This should be clearly stated so that any nurse, on reading the plan, can carry out all the prescribed care. Some health authorities encourage their district nurses to adopt the problem-solving approach and identify a nursing problem, prescribe the nursing care to be carried out, state who should carry out this care and evaluate the results of this care at regular intervals.

Some nurses continue to use the traditional progress records once they have acquired baseline information about their patients and identified their nursing and medical problems. There is a danger that this type of record will merely contain the nurse's observations of the patient and her routine actions and omit to say what is done in response to a problem. For continuity of care and adequate communication between fellow nurses and relief staff, it is important that once a nursing care problem has been recorded, the action taken, the progress of the problem or its resolution, should also be recorded.

IMPLEMENTATION

The third phase of the nursing process is the carrying out of nursing care as stated in the plan. On each visit by a member of the nursing team any relevant observations should be noted and reported to the district nursing sister. It is this nursing care given to patients by district nurses which is the substance of this book.

EVALUATION

Once the district nurse has decided upon the expected outcome or nursing goals then she has criteria established against which can be measured or compared the effects of the nursing care carried out. If the objectives have not been achieved then reassessment is necessary and the care plan changed accordingly. There is always a danger that the district nurse could put too much emphasis on the assessment stage and neglect the evaluation which is equally important. Hopefully this can be overcome by setting realistic goals in the first instance and stating a date when evaluation should take place. Progress notes are important in that they indicate the current status and progress of the patient when the nurse visits him but they must not replace evaluation – merely help the nurse to reconsider her care plan if the desired outcomes have not been achieved.

The stages of the nursing process are now the framework around which the new district nurse training is based.

The actual documentation used by district nurses for recording nursing assessments and care plans varies from healthy authority to health authority. The important thing is that it should be a problem-centred approach to planning nursing care.

BIBLIOGRAPHY

Long, R. (1981). *Systematic Nursing Care.* Faber and Faber, London.

McFarlane, J. and Castledine, G. (1982). *A Guide to the Practice of Nursing Using the Nursing Process.* Mosby-Year Book Limited, London.

Roper, N., Logan, W. and Tierney, A. (1980). *The Elements of Nursing.* Churchill Livingstone, Edinburgh.

Roper, N., Logan, W. and Tierney, A. (1981). *Learning to Use the Process of Nursing.* Churchill Livingstone, Edinburgh.

Roper, N., Logan, W. and Tierney, A. (1983). *Using a Model for Nursing.* Churchill Livingstone, Edinburgh.

Chapter Three

HOSPITAL DISCHARGES

THE NEED FOR CO-OPERATION

Nurses are aware of the need for the closest possible local co-operation between all the health services so that a pattern of co-ordinated patient care from home to hospital and back to the patient's home can be realised. Progressive patient care not only has important implications for individual hospitals, but also requires the development of a co-ordinated pattern of services on a community basis. Such a pattern should be based on the patient's needs and well-being, whether he is in hospital or in his home (DHSS, 1970).

There has been some research, not only into the needs of patients recently discharged from hospital, but also into how well these needs have been catered for by the domiciliary social and nursing services. Both Hockey (1968) and Skeet (1970) were concerned with hospital discharge procedures and the need for communication *with* patients and *between* professional staff so as to improve and achieve effective co-ordination of after-care services. In 1970 Hockey and Buttimore described an experiment to reduce surgical waiting lists by planned early discharge. In essence this meant effective collaboration between hospital and community staff in providing the necessary care to 'bridge the gap' between hospital and home.

Roberts (1975) tried to establish whether it was possible to measure the effectiveness of nursing after-care and at the same time to determine the conditions likely to influence the quality of such care. She aimed at discovering what kind of help people in various circumstances *believed* they needed and how it was provided. She found that there was a need for more systematic preparation for those leaving hospital, procedures to be put into action which considered the patient's capacity within the environment, and the consequent need for continuing care, taking into account the resources available. This does occur in specific areas of care:

(a) planned early discharge following surgery
(b) the elderly leaving geriatric wards
(c) maternity patients
(d) planned early discharge for coronary patients.

However, this specific planning does not always work on those occasions when patients are sent home earlier than expected.

EARLY DISCHARGE

Why are patients going home earlier? The early discharge of patients from surgical wards has become more common in recent years for various reasons.

The patient's benefit

Patients are now being mobilised earlier after surgery than they were 15 to 20 years ago. Doctors and nurses agree that remaining in bed carries more risk (deep vein thrombosis, chest infections, constipation and pressure sores) than mobilisation started the day after operation. Once the patient is free of any infusion, catheter or drainage tubes, the wound is healing well, and provided that progress is likely to be straightforward, then he might just as well be at home, supervised by his GP and the community nursing team. He can eat what he fancies and when he likes (unless he needs a special diet). No early waking; washing at leisure in his own bathroom; and the likelihood of a good night's rest in his own bed (without being disturbed by rattling trolleys, bedpans or noisy new admissions): all bonuses for early discharge.

At home he is surrounded by his family and can be involved in events going on around. He retains his authoritative role and is available to counsel, advise and direct, whereas in hospital he would tend to become isolated from family concerns. Wounds are likely to heal better at home where there is less risk of cross-infection.

Benefit to children

Much has been written about maternal deprivation and the need to prevent sick children from being separated from their mothers.

This previously unsatisfactory state of affairs has been improved by:

(a) allowing mothers to stay in hospital with their children
(b) carrying out more day-case surgery
(c) discharging children from hospital earlier
(d) paediatric domiciliary nursing schemes in some areas.

Children need familiar toys, surroundings and family faces – they tend to eat and drink more at home than when in hospital (see also p. 150).

The financial considerations of early discharge

In some cases it is cheaper to nurse someone at home rather than in hospital, where the National Health Service has to pay for his food, laundry, drugs, dressings, heating and staff salaries. At home the patient is cared for by the spouse or sibling, and food, laundry and heating bills are his responsibility. Drugs and dressings are obtained on prescription from his GP. The National Health Service only pays the cost of employing a district nurse to supervise care, do any dressings that are required and remove sutures on the appropriate day.

Reduction in the length of hospital waiting lists

One reason for early discharge is that this frees beds so that an increased number of patients may be admitted for cold surgery thus reducing hospital waiting lists. In Southampton a paediatric home-nursing scheme was started in conjunction with the Children's Hospital, and a waiting list which previously was two years for operations such as circumcision, herniorrhaphy and orchidopexy, was reduced to three weeks (Gow, 1977).

In selected patients early discharge after surgery can be beneficial, as well as allowing the district nurse a chance to practise more interesting procedures in her daily routine.

ASSESSING SUITABILITY FOR EARLY DISCHARGE

Planning and assessing are the key to any early discharge scheme:

(a) Operations which have a reasonably straightforward pre-operative, operative and postoperative course and a relatively low number of complications should be identified.

(b) Cases on the waiting list which can be dealt with on a short-stay basis should be selected, making any special arrangements for the nursing of them by the community nursing team after discharge. (Surgeons may need to re-evaluate surgical techniques, especially those of wound closure and drainage.) Arrangements may need to be made with the ambulance service for transport home.

(c) The patient's home environment will need to be evaluated as to its suitability for early discharge. Some surgeons like to discuss the possibility of early discharge with the patient when he is seen in the outpatients' department. He may then request (often *via* the community liaison sister) the district nurse to undertake a home assessment.

Community liaison

Effective liaison between hospital staff and the primary health care team members involved is essential.

GP to hospital doctor

It is essential that the patient's general practitioner informs the hospital consultant of any health problem or drugs the patient is taking, which could have an effect on early discharge. Many hospitals when informing the patient of admission to hospital now enclose a form to be completed by the GP and taken to hospital on admission. A 'post-discharge support request' form is often attached. Where this is relevant it should be filled in by the doctor or district nurse prior to admission. Where there is uncertainty about the patient's ability to care for himself after surgery, a home assessment visit by the district nurse can be arranged. She will inform the community liaison sister of the result of this visit and whether there are any problems or special needs.

District nurse to ward sister

If the district nurse is involved at this stage, she can ensure that the hospital staff know about any nursing treatment the patient may be receiving. This might include:

(a) cytamen injections for pernicious anaemia
(b) gold injections for rheumatoid arthritis
(c) adrenocorticotrophic hormone (ACTH) injections for multiple sclerosis or various other conditions
(d) dressings to ulcers or gangrenous toes.

It is highly unlikely that patients receiving cytamen, gold or ACTH would be considered suitable for early discharge. It is, however, useful if the ward sister is given details of the injection, and when the next one is due. This information may be given directly to the ward sister by telephone, or by contacting the community liaison sister or by letter taken to hospital by the patient.

Hospital doctor to GP

On discharge the GP should be informed either pre-discharge or soon after of what has been undertaken: in the case of surgery, what type of operation and the findings. Reports of any investigative procedure should also be provided. A discharge summary must be completed by the houseman and sent to the GP at the same time as the patient is discharged. In this way the GP knows what has been undertaken and, where relevant, what drugs the patient has been prescribed. It is important for the GP to know what has been said to the patient and/or relatives about the diagnosis, particularly if it involves a malignant condition.

Ward sister to district nurse

Details of any nursing care required by a patient being discharged early from hospital should be sent to the district nurse by the community liaison sister. It is her responsibility to visit the wards each day to find out who is being discharged and what care is needed. She then informs the relevant district nurse giving the patient's name, address, age, GP, the operation or condition treated, and the care needed. In one health district the ward sister completes a discharge form in quadruplicate; one copy is given to the patient to give to the district nurse when she calls; the second copy is sent by post to the district nurse with any extra details of the patient's condition (which he should not see) added; the third copy goes to the medical social work department, if home services are required; the final copy remains in the patient's case-note folder. The system varies throughout the country, but the basic principles remain the same, namely the giving of relevant information which may be summarised thus:

(a) Any nursing treatment required.
(b) The operation performed and the date when sutures are to be removed.
(c) Any injections required. These should include the drug,

strength, dose and the time or date when the next one is due.
(d) Any oral drugs which are to be taken.
(e) Any home services required such as home help, meals on wheels, attendance at a day hospital; together with confirmation of arrangements.
(f) Any equipment needed and whether or not this has been ordered.

It is important that before discharge the patient is given an adequate supply of drugs and dressings to last for at least three days until a prescription for more can be obtained from the GP. There is nothing more frustrating to the district nurse than to visit a newly discharged surgical patient at the weekend only to discover that the patient has not been given any dressings or lotions with which to pack an open wound. If the patient lives several miles out in the country, it can be time-consuming and expensive in petrol for her to obtain the necessary lotions and dressings. In some areas a central sterile supply department (CSSD) service is available for community staff, while in others everything has to be obtained on prescription.

Another aspect which should not be overlooked in the care of patients after early discharge is that primary health care team members should have copies of the detailed instructions which have been given to the patient (or parents in the case of a child). In some areas the patients are given a written sheet of instructions. If a new surgeon with different techniques and ideas about postoperative care is appointed, community nurses should be told of any changes in treatment which he might introduce.

Psychological support

The district nurse involved in the care of surgical patients, who have been discharged early from hospital, often has to give considerable emotional support. While in hospital the patient is surrounded by trained staff throughout the day and appears to be confident and self-assured, but once he has returned to his own home he frequently becomes unsure and often frightened. He may be scared that his wound will burst if he is sent home with sutures still in place and worries about coping with this eventuality. Alternatively, he (or she) may be distressed about the type of operation undergone, for example an ileostomy, mastectomy or amputation. The district nurse may have to give a great deal of reassurance and advice on how to manage any residual disability. In any step towards re-establishment of confidence she should make sure that the patient knows how to contact her.

DRESSINGS

When carrying out an aseptic dressing technique the district nurse must put into practice her hospital training; equally, she must be flexible enough to adapt it to the different situations in which she finds herself.

Central Sterile Supply Department (CSSD): As already mentioned, in some areas there is a central sterile supply department for dressings, which can be used by district nurses. The only items which must be obtained on prescription are the lotions and strapping. Other useful items provided by many CSSDs include mouth care packs, catheterisation packs, sterile ribbon gauze and receivers. This service is financed by the health authority at no cost to the patient.

Dressings obtained on prescription: In areas where this system works, the ward sister is asked to provide the patient with at least three days' supply of dressings so that he has time in which to arrange for a prescription to be collected from his GP and taken to the nearest chemist. Some patients are exempt from prescription charges but many are not, and the nurse should be as economical as possible. Some ill patients may be in financial difficulties. Ribbon gauze, sterile wool pads, strapping and lotions are all separate items on prescription and may not last long if the patient has an infected wound or varicose ulcer which needs daily dressings.

Sterilising instruments and receivers: This can be done in one of two ways if pre-sterilised items are not available. Boiling for 10 minutes in a large saucepan is a method still used by some district nurses who often instruct the patient how to do this so that all is ready when the nurse arrives. Many district nurses now use a special lotion to sterilise instruments and gallipots; instruments must be totally immersed for the prescribed length of time and the solution used once only.

Dressing techniques

The actual technique used varies in different parts of the country. Some district nurses use dressing forceps in the same way as in hospital. Soiled dressings are discarded either into thick paper bags or into newspaper, which should be burned if possible or else wrapped in more newspaper and placed in a plastic bag in the dustbin.

Another method is known as the Hampshire Dressing Aid (Fig. 3/1). This consists of a sterile plastic bag with an adhesive strip at the top and a pair of sterile disposable gloves for the nurse to wear when she does the dressing. She loosens the strapping securing the dressing and, with her hand in the polythene bag, removes the soiled dressing; at the same time she pulls the open end of the bag up over the hand holding the dressing, thus turning the bag inside out. The paper covering the adhesive strip is removed and the bag is attached to a near-by chair or table. The nurse then removes the plastic gloves from the paper containing them and puts them on. The paper itself can be used as a second sterile field or dressing towel. The patient's wound is cleaned, using the contents of the sterile dressing pack in the same way as in hospital. Most health authorities now provide their district nurses with sterile suture removal blades or CSSD suture removal packs. However, some nurses still have to sterilise forceps and scissors before removing sutures.

Because early discharge following surgery is on the increase the after-care and supervision of these patients is becoming a regular part of the district nurse's daily routine. She must plan her work so that clean dressings are carried out before the dirtier tasks and dirtier dressings that have to be done. In addition patients who have had open heart surgery to insert a pacemaker or to improve the blood supply to the heart are becoming more commonplace and need after-care from the district nurse.

HEART DISEASE

Over a quarter of a million people die of heart disease each year. In the 25 to 44 age-group, coronary thrombosis is the greatest single cause of death. It is said that about 3500 hospital beds are in use every day in Great Britain for the treatment of patients under 65 with this condition. Some of those suffering from a coronary thrombosis are cared for at home although the specialised care provided by coronary care units has led to a decrease of one-third in the coronary thrombosis death rate. Even so two out of five patients who have a coronary thrombosis die within the first hour.

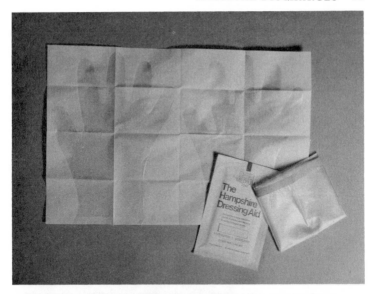

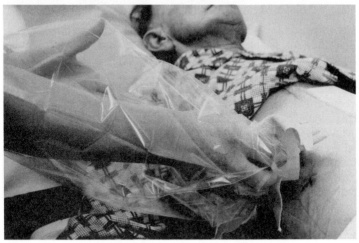

Fig. 3/1 The Hampshire Dressing Aid (*courtesy Surgikos Ltd*)

In places where sophisticated facilities are far distant, the GP may well decide to wait for 24 hours before transferring an elderly patient who has had a heart attack, to hospital.

The district nurse's involvement in coronary care is at first preventive. This aspect of her health education duties includes talking to patients about the risks to their health which their lifestyles and social habits can cause. These include cigarette smoking, obesity, lack of adequate exercise, stress, hypertension and possibly dietary factors (raised blood cholesterol and sugars).

Once the patient has had a coronary thrombosis, the nurse may visit him at home to administer analgesic injections, and to record pulse and blood pressure readings. In addition some nurses are also required to take an electrocardiograph reading to confirm the GP's provisional diagnosis.

The district nurse may well be asked to visit a patient who has been discharged from hospital after a coronary thrombosis. Reassurance is essential not only when the patient is in hospital but later when he is discharged into the more isolated home environment. It is then that symptoms, which are normally ignored, assume importance. This is when the district nurse comes in to comfort and reassure, explain his illness in simple terms, and encourage his rehabilitation. Naturally his family is included so that there is no breakdown in communication and no subsequent misinterpretation of instructions. Some hospitals provide a written check-list of instructions for the patient when he goes home. The district nurse also needs a copy of these instructions so that she can explain and reinforce them as necessary. She needs to be alert for any side-effects of anticoagulant therapy and report any signs of bleeding to the doctor. A regular check is made of blood pressure and pulse. It should not be overlooked that the nurse is also the main observer of the patient's behaviour and can therefore help his recovery by detecting any signs and symptoms of underlying emotional distress. Early referrals to the GP for treatment and reappraisal will aid rehabilitation and enable the patient to return to work sooner.

All patients discharged from hospital and referred to the district nurse for after-care need to be assessed carefully for nursing and other needs. In many cases only a few visits from the district nurse are needed. In others, especially in the case of elderly and handicapped patients, a more detailed assessment is needed and care planned to meet the individual's needs.

REFERENCES

DHSS (1970). *The State of the Public Health*. Report of the Chief Medical Officer 1970. HMSO, London.

Gow, M.A. (1977). Domiciliary paediatric care in Southampton. *Queen's Nursing Journal*, **19**, 7, 192 and 205.

Hockey, L. (1968). *Care in the Balance. A Study of Collaboration between Hospital and Community Services.* Queen's Institute of District Nursing, London.

Hockey, L. and Buttimore, A. (1970). *Co-operation in Patient Care. Studies of District Nurses Attached to Hospital and General Medical Practices.* Queen's Institute of District Nursing, London.

Roberts, I. (1975). *Discharged from Hospital.* Royal College of Nursing, London.

Skeet, M. (1970). *Home from Hospital.* Dan Mason Nursing Research Committee, London.

BIBLIOGRAPHY

Frazer, F.W. (ed) (1982). *Rehabilitation Within the Community.* Faber and Faber, London.

Simpson, J.E.P. and Levitt, R. (jt eds) (1981). *Going Home. A Guide for Helping the Patient on Leaving Hospital.* Churchill Livingstone, Edinburgh.

Chapter Four

THE DIABETIC PATIENT

PRIORITY OF THE DAY

As in hospital, the priority of the district nurse's working day is to diabetic patients needing insulin injections before breakfast. This means a visit between 8 a.m. and 9 a.m. There are two types of diabetic patient: the recently diagnosed diabetic, needing much help, advice and education on managing this condition in his life, and the patient who has had diabetes mellitus for many years, possibly now suffering from side-effects of the disease. There may be defective vision coupled with an inability to draw up an insulin injection accurately. This necessitates a visit from the district nurse to check the urinalysis, give the insulin injection and sort out any problems, for instance, a home visit by the chiropodist may need to be arranged because the progressive nature of the disease means that the patient is no longer able to attend the chiropody sessions at the local health centre. The district nurse should be aware of the hazards of infection in wounds of the lower limbs, and the rapidity with which gangrene can set in where the circulation is deficient. Reassessment and speedy referral for medical advice are important in caring for diabetics.

THE NEWLY DIAGNOSED DIABETIC

The diabetic requiring insulin

The district nurse may be asked by the community liaison sister at the local district general hospital to visit a recently diagnosed diabetic discharged from hospital 'fully stabilised and capable of giving himself insulin injections'. The 'protected' environment in hospital, where the diet is calculated and prepared for the patient and where disposable syringes are pre-sterilised and ready for use, is a far cry from home. The 'stabilised diabetic state' can become 'unstabilised' as the patient reverts to his normal more energetic routine. The district nurse must reinforce the instructions given during the patient's stay in hospital concerning the signs and symptoms of hypoglycaemia – the need to carry lumps of sugar or glucose sweets; an identification card stating his name, address, GP's name and telephone number; insulin dosage and instructions on how to help if he is found in a coma. The insulin dose may need to be reduced or more carbohydrate may be needed in the diet to compensate for that burnt up during exercise or work. Liaison with the patient's GP and consultant is imperative at this time.

The first visit

Do not worry if the first visit to the home of a newly diagnosed diabetic is prolonged. There are so many aspects of care to consider in addition to emergency instructions, dietary advice, supervision of urine testing for sugar and ketones, and drawing up and injecting the insulin. Various manufacturers produce diabetic education booklets which help to reinforce the district nurse's teaching at this time.

Dietary advice

Most newly diagnosed diabetics are visited routinely by the hospital dietician prior to discharge. The patient, armed with diet sheet and booklet or list of foods each containing 10 grams (g) of carbohydrate, is ready to return home. The district nurse may need to explain it all again to the diabetic and his family if they are unsure or forgetful of the dietician's instructions. Consequently it is important that the district nurse liaises with the dietician and keeps up-to-date with new trends in diabetic dietary control. All diabetics need to watch the type as well as the amount of carbohydrate eaten. Refined carbohydrate such as cakes, pastries, sugary foods and puddings should be avoided and wholemeal bread, vegetables, fruit and high fibre foods encouraged. A reduction in fatty foods is also recommended with the ultimate aim of preventing the diabetic from becoming overweight or getting long-term complications associated with the condition.

The nurse must ensure that her diabetic patient understands *why* he should always carry sugar in case of an insulin reaction. He must be able to recognise the signs of hypoglycaemia: shaking, trembling, sweating, hunger, headache, pins and needles in the tongue and lips, palpitations, slurring of the speech, and double vision. Later signs that relatives should be aware of include confusion, behavioural changes and coma. The danger times are before lunch and during the night. Most insulin-dependent diabetics have now been changed over to U100 insulin and have been given new syringes, a U100 dosage card and explanatory leaflets. The district nurse must be extra careful when visiting a newly referred diabetic who might still be using the old U20, U40 or U80 strengths.

Care of syringes and needles

Sterilisation and storage of syringes and needles are other aspects of the teaching process. Each nurse tends to have her own method of storage. A small Pyrex butter dish with a lid is as good as any. The dish and lid can be boiled weekly as can the syringe and needles. Industrial methylated spirits, only available on prescription, should be used to soak the syringe and needles in between the weekly boiling routine. It is important to operate the plunger of the syringe several times to remove all traces of spirit before drawing up the insulin. Plastic disposable syringes and needles can be *bought* from the chemist or British Diabetic Association but cannot be obtained on prescription. Diabetics should always have at least two syringes, one spare in case of loss or damage. Portable spirit-proof syringe cases are available under the National Health Service but the plastic 'Insulin-User's Case' is not and has to be ordered from Hypoguard Ltd (see p. 49) or the British Diabetic Association. Diabetics are exempt from prescription charges, but they must have an exemption certificate issued by the Family Practitioner Committee and obtained through their GP. This has to be renewed every three years.

Urinalysis

It is advisable for the new diabetic to test the urine for the presence of sugar before meals or as directed by his physician. The patient should receive clear instructions to pass urine to empty the bladder about half an hour before testing, so that the tested specimen is fresh and has not been in the bladder for several hours. The nurse should supervise this testing on her first visits. If the patient is using Clinitest tablets as urine testing reagents, the district nurse must stress the importance of keeping the lid tightly screwed or the tablets will absorb moisture from the air, making the test result inaccurate. Other similar tests are those using plastic strips impregnated with a reagent which changes colour when dipped into a specimen of urine if sugar is present. Once the new diabetic is fully stabilised such frequent urine testing may not be necessary. Many physicians prefer blood glucose monitoring as a better method of achieving accurate control of the diabetic condition (see p. 46).

The drawing up and giving of insulin

Insulin should be injected 15 to 20 minutes before breakfast and other meals as directed by the doctor. The cloudy types of insulin should be shaken before use but the clear types should not be shaken. Before leaving hospital the patient will have been taught how to give himself insulin injections, but the district nurse should make sure that he is confident in carrying this out.

The role of the district nurse

Few diseases demand as much patient participation in therapy as diabetes. Nearly all diabetics must manage their disease by themselves in everyday life. This places a different responsibility on the district nurse, namely that of making the patient a knowledgeable, willing manager of his own care. Before the district nurse discharges a newly diagnosed diabetic from her care she should apply a few basic rules. The patient must have:

- Full understanding of the disease and the need for therapy
- Ability to monitor the control of his condition by either urinalysis or blood glucose monitoring
- Awareness of the need to seek medical advice if test results record a persistently high sugar content with signs of a high blood sugar such as excessive thirst, urination or fatigue
- A concept of varying injection sites so as to prevent the changes in the fatty tissues which can interfere with the absorption of insulin
- Ability to draw up the prescribed dose of insulin and inject it correctly
- Dietary control: the need for a diet reduced in carbohydrate and fatty foods but high in fibre content and taken regularly
- Adaptation of lifestyle to fit a diabetic regime
- Knowledge of how to deal with a hypoglycaemic reaction or illness
- Knowledge of the need for daily foot care (Table 4/1)

- Knowledge of how to contact the district nurse if problems arise.

Table 4/1 Dos and don'ts in foot care for diabetics

Dos	Don'ts
Wear well-fitting shoes	No soaking in hot water
Wash feet daily and dry thoroughly	No cutting of corns or toenails if the eyesight is poor
Inspect feet daily	
Report suspicious lesions immediately	No walking barefoot
Have regular chiropody treatment	No tight stockings or garters
	No hot-water bottles

The hospital nurse sees diabetics who are acutely ill, such as those needing surgical operations; those in a state of hypoglycaemic or hyperglycaemic coma and those suffering from acute infections or diabetic gangrene. The district nurse has a less dramatic, but equally important role in caring for diabetics – that of educator and enabler.

The diabetic controlled by tablets

The idea that oral treatment allows more freedom of action and less need for supervision of the diabetes is not only false, but is positively dangerous. Even mild, maturity-onset diabetes must be properly controlled and the closest attention paid to diet and weight. Every diabetic must know his ideal weight and attempt to keep to it. Often the taking of oral anti-diabetic agents is an excuse for over-eating.

The greatest danger of these drugs is uncontrolled hypoglycaemia. Although it occurs less often than with insulin treatment, it can continue for some days and even cause death, particularly in older patients. The district nurse must ensure that her patients know the signs and symptoms and what to do if hypoglycaemia occurs. Occasionally side-effects occur when patients are taking these tablets. The district nurse should alert herself to this possibility.

Tolbutamide can cause headaches, indigestion and decreased tolerance to alcohol in some individuals. Jaundice has also been reported.

Chlorpropamide may cause digestive upsets, dizziness, headaches, rashes, general malaise, foul taste in the mouth, jaundice and even bone marrow malfunction.

The diabetic controlled by diet alone

Loss of weight for many obese, maturity-onset diabetics can mean the return to normal blood sugar levels without the need for any drug therapy either by mouth or by injection. This type of diabetic should be given a reducing diet. The district nurse may be asked to visit once a week to weigh the patient, test the urine for sugar and generally supervise the diet.

THE CHILD DIABETIC

Management of a child diabetic differs from that of an adult. This is partly because the child will certainly require insulin injections and because he will need minute modifications in his diet and treatment to avoid hypoglycaemic attacks, and to allow for his size and growth spurts. Once the parents have got over the shock of their child being diabetic it is essential that they, as well as the young patient, fully understand his diabetic regime and injection technique (Fig. 4/1). One of the greatest difficulties is relating diet to exercise. If a child is extra active he will need more food, preferably before and during extra activity, as the diabetic child absorbs glucose after exercise with less dependence on insulin.

School dinners can usually be modified by increasing the amount of vegetables and reducing potatoes, and by substituting fresh fruit or cheese and biscuits for the pudding. Some diabetic children may prefer to go home for dinner or take a packed lunch to school.

THE BLIND DIABETIC

Blindness comes as a shock to anyone and to the diabetic it comes as a double blow. Because of tactile sensitivity loss and circulatory impairment, the diabetic may have more difficulty learning to use Braille, moving around or keeping up with a job. Worst of all, blindness interferes with two activities essential to the diabetic's

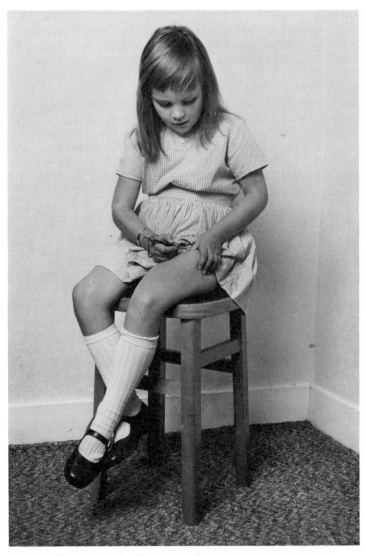

Fig. 4/1 Girl injecting insulin (*courtesy British Diabetic Association*)

existence, namely the giving of his own insulin injections and the monitoring of his condition.

Many diabetics are strongly motivated towards independence and will be able to overcome this further handicap providing they have a relative to check their urinalysis and the setting of a pre-set

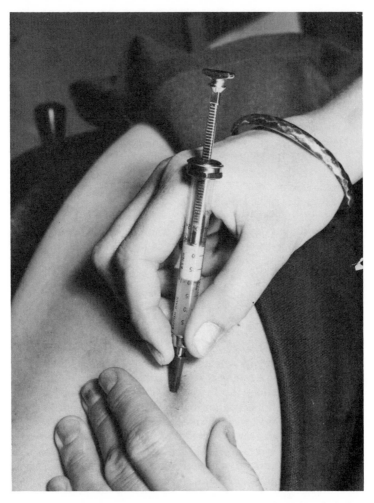

Fig. 4/2 The 'Click/Count' syringe (*courtesy British Diabetic Association*)

syringe every one to two days. Another available syringe is the Click/Count Syringe (Fig. 4/2). Each click corresponds to one mark on the syringe so that the patient can both feel and hear the measurement. The use of the syringe should be supervised in the first instance by the district nurse.

There are still many diabetics who are unable to cope when their vision is impaired and if they live alone then they must be visited daily by the district nurse. Often elderly relatives are not confident enough to shoulder this responsibility or may have failing vision themselves.

Other help to registered 'blind' or 'partially sighted' people includes:

Rehabilitation and vocational assessment at the Royal National Institute for the Blind at Torquay
Help from the blind person's disablement resettlement officer at the local Job Centre
Home teachers for the blind
Braille books
Guide dogs (and exemption from a dog licence)
Supplementary benefits
Reduction in cost of a black and white television licence
Loans of tape-recorders and tapes of books from the RNIB
Free postage on articles for the blind.

THE DIABETIC SUFFERING FROM GANGRENE OF THE LOWER LIMB

Arteriosclerosis is a common condition in elderly diabetics. Peripheral neuropathy which makes the patient insensitive to pain and injury, is also a common complication of diabetes mellitus and means that a patient can injure his limbs without feeling pain. Tissues saturated in sugar are an ideal medium for the growth and proliferation of most bacteria and so a moist gangrene often occurs.

The infected area must be dressed daily. It may be for this reason that the patient is referred initially to the care of the district nurse. The diabetes must be stabilised and the patient may have to commence insulin injections. If the gangrene cannot be controlled he may ultimately have to undergo an amputation of a toe, a foot or even a leg. The district nurse will then be concerned with the

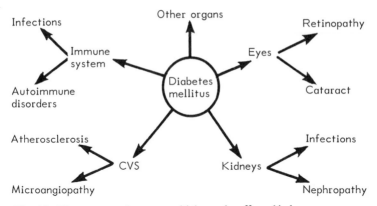

Fig. 4/3 The organs and systems which may be affected in long-term diabetes

rehabilitation of an amputee as well as supervising his diabetic therapy.

If staffing levels permit, the ideal situation would include the regular visiting of all diabetics by either a health visitor or district nurse attached to the diabetic clinic. In this way the nurse can check that treatment is understood and being followed and also note the early signs of complications. Figure 4/3 shows how complications may arise in long-term diabetes.

DIAGNOSTIC TESTS FOR DIABETES

Glycosuria suggests diabetes. High blood glucose levels indicate diabetes in anyone displaying other symptoms of the disease. A glucose tolerance test confirms the diagnosis and indicates the best method of treatment.

Glucose tolerance test

Some GPs refer their patients to the pathological laboratory technician for this investigation, while others arrange for it to be carried out in the health centre or the patient's home by the district nurse. It is a lengthy procedure, taking a total of about 2½ hours to perform and not all district nurses have the time available to do this. Obviously it is best done in the morning so that the patient can fast naturally during the previous night and so that specimens can be rapidly sent off to the laboratory.

Instructions to the patient

1. Eat your normal diet for the week preceding the test. Do not restrict carbohydrates.
2. Eat or drink nothing after 8 p.m. on the night before the test and have no breakfast or cup of tea before the test.
3. The nurse should always explain the test itself and why it is necessary.

Equipment

5 × 2ml syringes with 21 s.w.g. needles
5 × blood glucose specimen bottle (yellow in colour) containing fluoride oxalate
5 × urine specimen bottles
50g of glucose in 200ml water
Medical wipes
Tourniquet or sphygmomanometer and cuff
Clock
Request form

Procedure

1. Ask the patient to empty his bladder and collect a fasting urine specimen for testing for glucose. Label it 'fasting specimen'.
2. Take 2ml of blood by venepuncture and place in a yellow bottle. Label it 'fasting specimen'.
3. Ensure that the glucose is properly dissolved then ask the patient to drink all the glucose solution.
4. Further blood and urine specimens are collected at 30-minute intervals, that is 30, 60, 90 and 120 minutes after consuming the glucose.
5. Label the specimens with the patient's name, date and time. Store in the refrigerator and despatch to the laboratory as soon as possible after they are all obtained.
6. Advise the patient to make an appointment to see his doctor within the next week.

Clinical note: Fasting venous blood glucose levels of 7.2mmol/litre (130mg/100ml) or more with failure to return to fasting levels in two hours are diagnostic of diabetes mellitus.

Routine blood glucose monitoring

Two main types of reagent strip are now available commercially and can be used to monitor blood glucose levels. The medical opinion today is that blood glucose monitoring is more efficient in achieving diabetic stability than urine testing alone. Better diabetic control reduces the risk of the long-term complications of the condition. Many diabetics have bought their own glucometers to measure the readings accurately; others rely on the reagent strips and compare the results with a colour chart. The district nurse should be aware of new developments in this field.

Dextrostix

1. These must be stored away from light, moisture or excessive heat to prevent loss of sensitivity. Individual strips in foil are best.
2. Avoid handling the test end of the strip.
3. Do not lay the reagent strip on a table surface or absorbent towel – use a clean sheet of paper.
4. Ensure the lighting is good for reading the strip.
5. Explain the procedure to the patient and ask him to wash his hands under a warm tap but not to use soap.
6. Assemble the equipment:
   Dextrostrip – check the expiry date
   Colour chart
   Lancet or autolet
   Tissues
   Wash bottle containing water
   Watch with a second hand
7. Compare the Dextrostrip reagent area with 'O' block on the colour chart and do not use if there is a colour variant.
8. Prick the patient's thumb or finger using a lancet or autolet.
9. Apply a large drop of the capillary blood so that the whole reagent area on the printed side of the strip is covered. Insufficient blood will lead to inaccurate readings.
10. Wait exactly 60 seconds.
11. Quickly wash off the blood with a sharp stream of water from the wash bottle.
12. Read immediately (within 1 or 2 seconds) by holding the strip close to the colour chart.
13. Record the readings in the patient's nursing notes.

For a more accurate reading of the Dextrostix, a *glucometer* (Fig. 4/4) can be used to measure glucose values between

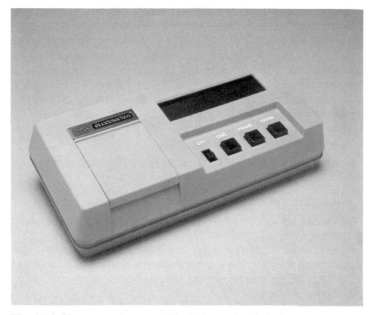

Fig. 4/4 A Glucometer (*courtesy Miles Laboratories Limited (Ames Division)*)

0–22.2mmol/litre. It is also useful to those many diabetics with impaired colour vision who could not accurately use the colour chart with the Dextrostix strips. The instrument should be calibrated weekly according to the instructions to ensure accuracy. It is a portable, battery-operated instrument.

Operation of glucometer

1. Switch to 'on'.
2. Press the time button and a buzzer sounds. This is the signal to apply blood or a control solution (when calibrating) to the Dextrostix reagent strip pad.
3. A second buzzer sounds after 60 seconds countdown on the digital display.
4. Immediately wash the reagent strip; blot with a tissue and insert into the test chamber strip guide.
5. Press the read button and the test result is clearly displayed.

Glycemie Stixs (BM-test Glycemie 20–800)

As with Dextrostix only fresh capillary blood from the finger or ear lobe should be used for the test. The test strip should be protected against humidity and direct sunlight and so the test strip vial must be closed with the desiccant stopper immediately after removal of a test strip.

Procedure

1. Check the test strip has not changed colour and is not out of date.
2. Prepare the patient and prick his thumb in the same way as for Dextrostix.
3. Apply one drop of blood to the test patch. Do not spread over the surface.
4. After exactly one minute, wipe off the blood with a dry cotton wad or tissue.
5. Leave for a further minute and match the colour with the chart on the container. When values exceed 13.3mmol/l (240mg/100ml) compare the colours two minutes after wiping.

BIBLIOGRAPHY

Farquhar, J. W. (1981). *The Diabetic Child*, 3rd edition. Churchill Livingstone, Edinburgh.

Farquhar, J. W. (1982). *Diabetes in Your Teens*. Churchill Livingstone, Edinburgh.

Guthrie, D. W. and Guthrie, R. A. (1982). *Nursing Management of Diabetes Mellitus*, 2nd edition. Mosby-Year Book Limited, London.

Tattersall, R. (1981). *Diabetes: A Practical Guide for Patients on Insulin*. Churchill Livingstone, Edinburgh.

EQUIPMENT NOTE

Hypoguard Limited, Dock Lane, Melton, Woodbridge, Suffolk IP12 1PE.

Chapter Five

THE PATIENT WITH LEG ULCERS

The patient suffering from leg ulceration is familiar to the district nurse, and caring for these people takes up much of her time.

CAUSES OF LEG ULCERATION

Common pre-disposing factors in the development of leg ulcers include: increased venous pressure; trauma; infection; arterial insufficiency and obesity.

Rarer causes include the gumma of syphilis, malignant neoplasms, artefact injuries, cutaneous tuberculosis and hypertension.

If the district nurse understands the reasons why venous ulceration develops not only will she be able to apply the principles of treatment but she will also be able to advise patients on prevention.

The development of leg ulcers due to increased venous pressure (Figs. 5/1; 5/2)

Damage to deep veins: Damage to, and incompetence of, the valves of the deep and communicating veins usually follow a deep vein thrombosis, after which a process of re-canalisation occurs to re-establish the flow of blood in the vein. During this process valves are destroyed and a system of re-canalised veins without valves established. This causes a backflow from the deep to the superficial veins resulting in raised pressure in the latter. At a later stage varicosities can develop. Initially, although the capillaries are damaged, oedema, reactive fibrosis and lymphatic obstruction occur and the limb appears swollen, with poorly oxygenated tissues. An injury or infection may precipitate the development of an ulcer or it can happen spontaneously.

For the patient who has had a deep vein thrombosis, the district

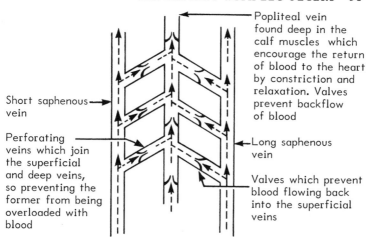

Popliteal vein
found deep in the
calf muscles which
encourage the return
of blood to the heart
by constriction and
relaxation. Valves
prevent backflow
of blood

Short saphenous
vein

Perforating
veins which join
the superficial
and deep veins,
so preventing the
former from being
overloaded with
blood

Long saphenous
vein

Valves which prevent
blood flowing back
into the superficial
veins

Fig. 5/1 Normal venous circulation in the lower leg

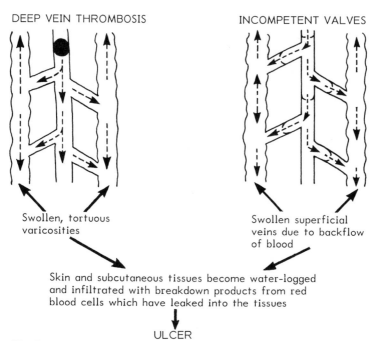

DEEP VEIN THROMBOSIS

INCOMPETENT VALVES

Swollen, tortuous
varicosities

Swollen superficial
veins due to backflow
of blood

Skin and subcutaneous tissues become water-logged
and infiltrated with breakdown products from red
blood cells which have leaked into the tissues

ULCER

Fig. 5/2 Failure in the venous circulation leading ultimately to an ulcer

nurse should advise the wearing of well-fitting elastic stockings. This helps to reduce the venous pressure in superficial veins and so prevent capillary damage and swelling, with subsequent development of leg ulcers.

Damage to superficial veins: Superficial varicose veins can develop as a result of valvular incompetence in the superficial veins and, perhaps, in some communicating veins. Oedema is much less marked and though ulceration can occur, it is rarer than the post-thrombotic type of ulceration. Treatment of varicosities either by sclerosing injections or by surgery reduces the incidence of this type of venous ulcer. Depending on the surgeon's practice the nurse may need to encourage compression bandaging for six weeks following surgery or injections (Fig. 5/3). Foot exercises need to be encouraged: they will have been taught by a physiotherapist.

PREVENTION OF LEG ULCERATION

The early treatment of varicosities and the wearing of compression bandages or stockings following a deep vein thrombosis have been mentioned. Prevention of the initial thrombosis in at-risk patients is also important, but is more of a medical than a nursing problem except when it comes to the early mobilisation of surgical patients.

Preventive advice to those at risk of developing varicose ulcers

- Avoid standing and, whenever possible, take a few steps
- Do not sit with legs crossed at the ankle as this prevents venous return
- Do no sit with legs elevated exerting pressure on calf muscles
- Wear lace-up shoes, not slippers, and if the feet perspire change to another pair of similar shoes
- Sit normally but move the ankles up and down as often as possible
- Walk as much as possible, within your limitations
- Raise the foot of the bed and if possible lie on the raised bed for half an hour during the day
- Do not sit too close to the fire and only bath at night time because a hot bath in the morning and the heat from the fire both tend to engorge the superficial veins with blood
- Wear supportive stockings or bandages as either a preventive or post-healing measure

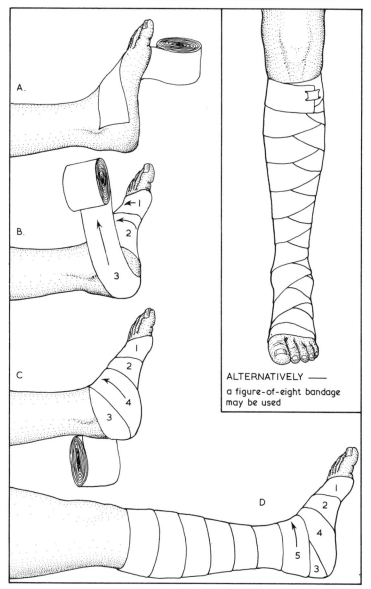

A.

B.

C.

ALTERNATIVELY ——

a figure-of-eight bandage
may be used

D

Fig. 5/3 The application of a compression (support) bandage

ASSESSMENT

The aspects of assessment for particular attention on the first visit are:

1. Whether the patient lives alone or has relatives who help with the housework, laundry and cooking, or whether a home help is needed and would be appreciated.
2. The degree of mobility and problems, if any, with personal hygiene and toilet. Referral to the community occupational therapist should be considered.
3. The type of house and its accessibility. For instance, an arthritic patient with varicose ulcers would find stairs difficult ordinarily, but if the ankles are stiff and fixed due to the effects of the ulcers the problem becomes acute. The bed might well have to be moved downstairs and a commode borrowed. The possibility of rehousing in ground floor accommodation should be investigated after discussion with the patient.
4. Diet. This should be discussed with the patient with the nurse advising on foods containing iron and vitamin C, both of which are needed to encourage wound healing. Later the nurse may discuss with the general practitioner the advisability of a haemoglobin test as patients with leg ulcers are often anaemic and anaemia delays healing. This vicious circle can be broken by the provision of additional iron and a nourishing diet. Meals on wheels can be valuable at this time.
5. Assessment of the amount of exercise which the patient takes each day and the type of work done (if not retired). Employment which involves standing behind counters, lathes or desks is conducive to the development of increased venous pressure as the patient's calf muscle pump is not being sufficiently utilised and the blood flow stagnates.
6. Recording of blood pressure and pulse rate, and urinalysis should be carried out as both hypertension and diabetes can cause leg ulcers.
7. The skin should be examined for signs of injury, infection or allergy. An ulcer can be measured either with a tape measure or by tracing the area of the lesion on to transparent film. The latter method gives the patient and nurse the satisfaction of checking the healing process. A wound swab should be taken and sent to the laboratory for microscopy, culture and

sensitivity. Any infection discovered is usually treated with systemic antibiotics as topical preparations may cause allergic contact dermatitis of the surrounding skin.

TREATMENT

Before healing and granulation can occur, any infection must be treated, the ulcer cleaned and any slough removed. Infected ulcers which are discharging copiously should be dressed daily as the purulent discharges can further irritate the surrounding skin. Preparations which are used for cleaning dirty ulcers and promoting granulation include: eusol (with or without liquid paraffin); Unguentum Merck; Aserbine cream or lotion; Debrisan; Varidase solution; and hydrogen peroxide.

Medication for the lesion

The ulcer can be dressed in various ways but tulle gras is popular. However, medicated tulle such as Sofra-Tulle and Fucidin Intertulle, should be used with care because of the possibility of contact dermatitis.

Simple medicaments impregnated into cotton bandages can be applied to the limb to help control its skin sensitivity, relieve itching and treat infection. Various bandages are available and should be chosen according to the condition of the skin:

A simple zinc paste bandage for straightforward varicose ulcers
An ichthammol paste bandage for weeping eczemas as well as ulcers
A coal-tar paste bandage for varicose ulcers surrounded by a dry itchy eczema
A zinc paste bandage impregnated with iodochloro-hydroxyquinoline 1% for infected lesions.

If the ulcer is raw, deep or painful, a small piece of tulle gras (the exact size of the ulcer) can be applied over it, but otherwise no dressing is needed under the paste bandage. Some nurses apply 1% gentian violet to the unstable skin around the ulcer to protect it from pus and exudate.

Application of a paste bandage

The patient's leg must be kept raised to prevent the accumulation of oedema while the dressing and paste bandage are applied. The foot is maintained at right-angles and the bandage applied gently and evenly from the base of the toes to the tibial tuberosity, ensuring that the heel is included. One method, other than the traditional spiral bandaging, is to take the bandage round the leg and then fold it back at each turn, the fold being at the side of the leg. This facilitates removal as cutting is unnecessary because the folds can be gently pulled back, as long as the bandage remains soft.

An absorbent pressure pad can be made over the ulcer itself either by applying six to eight folds of the bandage to and fro over it, or else by placing a piece of foam over the ulcer prior to the application of the pressure bandage.

Compression bandaging (Fig. 5/3)

The aim of compression bandaging is to minimise fluid leakage into the tissues and to maintain venous flow when the calf muscle pump is at rest. Support is provided by a paste bandage which also protects the skin and serves as a dressing for the ulcer to prevent infection. Further compression can be provided by the application of another bandage such as a blue- or red-line elasticated bandage, over the paste bandage, or it may be applied by itself. Other types of bandage which may be used include an elastocrêpe bandage which can be washed and used a second time or a slightly adhesive bandage, Lestreflex, which adheres and adjusts to the limb contours as the body heat warms the lead oleate in the bandage. This latter bandage cannot be used a second time. A simple crêpe bandage is not satisfactory as it does not allow sufficient compression.

Application of a compression bandage is important so that even pressure is applied the length of the lower leg. The bandage should reach from the base of the metatarsal to the tibial tuberosity and include the heel. If the bandage is applied correctly it will feel comfortable to the wearer. If the patient complains of pain the bandage must be re-applied.

OTHER ASPECTS OF TREATMENT

Dressing changes

If the ulcer is large and 'wet', the dressing and compression bandages can be changed twice a week, but the more usual regime is a weekly or fortnightly visit. If there is excessive discharge the patient can place an absorbent pad over the leaking area and change that daily without interfering with the bandage.

Regular daily exercise

Many varicose ulcer patients are elderly and incapacitated. For those who are able to do so, a daily walk is recommended to keep the calf muscle pump in action. If they are employed in work which involves standing, patients should shift from foot to foot and move the feet individually up and down regularly. If sitting is unavoidable then ankle movements, keeping the toes in contact on the floor, should be encouraged. For those who are able, walking up and down stairs is useful.

Many of the district nurse's patients lack motivation because of personality, health, domestic or social problems. It is all too easy to 'give up' and abandon attempts at walking; the ankle then becomes fixed and the patient retires to a chair in a depressed state of mind and tends towards self-neglect. Attendance at a varicose ulcer clinic often helps, for the patient meets others similarly placed or even worse than he is; he is thus able to face the fact that there are others also who have to cope with what to him is a miserable condition. Such contact can help to improve his outlook as well as providing social support. Physiotherapy may help to mobilise a stiffened ankle joint.

Bedrest and elevation

Short periods of bedrest with the foot of the bed elevated on blocks are beneficial, but prolonged bedrest should be discouraged as it can result in further complications.

After-care

Once the ulcer is healed the patient should continue to wear supportive bandages during the day for about six weeks to help toughen the skin. After this an elastic stocking should be worn. Adequate exercise remains vital and the district nurse should remind her patient about this before discharging him from her care. The early reporting of further injuries to the fragile healed ulcer area should also be emphasised.

The district nurses who run varicose ulcer clinics receive much satisfaction from seeing really large leg ulcers heal without the patient having to be admitted to hospital.

BIBLIOGRAPHY

Camp, R. (1977). Leg ulcers. *Nursing Times*, 25 August.

Fry, L. (1973). *Dermatology – An Illustrated Guide*. Update, London.

Wilson, D. (1977). Horses for courses at Staines. *Journal of Community Nursing*, 18 August.

Chapter Six

DYING AT HOME

The majority of people die in old age. Consequently there is a greater likelihood of prolonged infirmity and sickness before death which may happen at home. The disappearance of the extended family and the reduction in size of family units now mean that less people die at home, because there are no relatives to care for them. The district nurse visits most terminally ill patients registered with the practice to which she is attached. While there has been an increase in units which specialise in continuing care, it is felt that it would be beneficial to have a unit in each health district. This would enable a combined service with community nurses and the GP providing pain and symptom control clinics with in-patient facilities. Many areas do employ Macmillan nurses who are able to offer extra support for patients, relatives and community nurses in this area of patient care.

CONSIDERATIONS BEFORE THE FIRST VISIT

Caring for a dying patient can be a physical and emotional strain on all involved, including the nurse. It should be remembered that nurses themselves need support and counselling at times and the availability of a colleague with whom they can talk and express their fears and problems can be a great help and relief. The 'treatment and cure' model of nurse training is giving way to the 'caring' model which involves the use of the nursing process and a problem-solving approach to nursing care. No longer is dying considered to be a 'failure' but rather a challenge to nurses to ensure that the care that they give improves the quality of life remaining to the patient so that he dies peacefully.

Before visiting her patient for the first time the district nurse must know whether the patient and family are aware of the diagnosis and prognosis. While the actual telling is the doctor's responsibility it is often the nurse or family who are faced with the question 'Am I dying?' It is important that a question such as this should not be brushed aside. Each nurse develops her own way of coping with such situations and much will depend on her knowledge of her patient and how he will react to being told. The family may have decided that he should not be told. There is the ethical problem 'Should he be told?' Most patients probably guess that something is wrong by their decreasing strength and physical capacities together with possible changes in the attitudes of their family and care-givers. For all these reasons it *is* important for the district nurse to find out before visiting the patient whether he or his family know that he is dying. It may be later, when reassessing the needs of the patient and the family, that the district nurse decides that they need to know the severity of the illness. She should then discuss this with the GP.

THE FIRST VISIT

As already described the first visit is one of assessing and planning. In the case of the dying, particular note should be made of:

(a) the effectiveness of the drugs
(b) any particularly distressing symptoms
(c) the condition of skin and pressure areas
(d) the need for any nursing aids and equipment to make the patient more comfortable
(e) any problems relating to the urinary tract or bowel such as incontinence of urine or faeces, frequency of micturition, dysuria or constipation
(f) any disturbance of normal sleep pattern and/or night confusion
(g) the ability of the patient to care for himself in washing, feeding and toileting.

After having talked with the patient and answered any questions, the district nurse can discuss his needs and a possible plan of nursing care. The aim should be to maintain a normal pattern and not remove responsibilities and directive powers. The mother will wish to be involved and consulted about the running of the house, and the father will want to be asked his advice about any decisions. If a lady normally has her hair set each week the nurse should try and arrange for her to have this done at home.

Flexibility is important when planning care, and as evaluation is virtually a continuous process because the patient's needs may be changing from day to day, so the plan of care will need to be changed.

It is useful for the nurse to learn of her patient's religious beliefs. This can be done as she is filling in personal details on the Nursing History Record. From this she can casually ask whether the priest or minister visits. It is helpful if the nurse is aware of the depth of her patient's beliefs so that spiritual help may be provided if this is his wish and so that the rituals and customs of the dying person's religion may be observed at the appropriate time. The Roman Catholic may wish for the Sacrament of the Sick. When a Jew dies his body must not be touched and the Rabbi must be called.

On this first visit the district nurse should talk to the relatives who will be bearing the brunt of the care. She can advise on how to care for the patient and help them to cope generally.

PROBLEMS WHEN CARING FOR THE DYING
Pain

If pain is a problem the important thing is the establishing of freedom from pain without over-sedation so that it interferes with his relationships with others. Individual reaction to pain is complex as it is influenced by genetics, culture, past experience, emotion, anxiety, religion and many other personal characteristics. Pain may bring about emotional and psychological changes in even the most well-balanced patient, resulting in his becoming withdrawn, sullen, anxious, depressed and even aggressive.

The district nurse needs to be aware of this when she makes her initial assessment of her patient and his needs. The most important step in the nursing care of her patient is to listen carefully to what he says. In this way she can understand and assuage his fears and anxieties, and clear up misconceptions about the illness, treatment and any related factors. Knowledge helps to dispel fear and increases confidence in those caring for him.

The actual prescription of analgesics is the GP's responsibility. However, the district nurse should take time to make sure that the patient and relatives understand the importance of giving the right dosage at the right time. For patients with chronic pain, regular four-hourly analgesia has been shown to be the most effective. Many doctors prefer to start the patient on a low dose of morphia for moderate pain as this is easier to adjust. The aim is to titrate the level of analgesia against the patient's pain, gradually increasing the dose until the patient is pain free. To achieve this the next dose is given before the total effect of the previous one has worn off, and therefore before the patient feels it is necessary. If this regime is continued the patient no longer fears the onset of pain. A useful recently manufactured analgesic is slow-release morphia tablets (MST) which need to be taken only 12-hourly.

Most terminally ill patients can tolerate oral analgesia until a few days before they die when nausea or inability to swallow become a problem. Sublingual buprenorphine (Temgesic) may help in this instance. Alternatively many analgesic drugs can be provided in a suppository form, e.g. morphine, dextromoramide (Palfium) and oxycodone pectinate. The nurse may have to revert to injections in the last few days in order to achieve pain control and the patient is often emaciated by this time. Injection sites should be varied to prevent soreness and if the prescribed analgesic is diamorphine it can be given subcutaneously. The use of a syringe driver is helpful both in achieving freedom from pain and in avoiding four-hourly injections. The district nurse is responsible for the accurate recording of the administration of controlled drugs. When the patient dies she should adhere to the health authority's policy for their safe disposal.

Bone metastases

In disseminated carcinoma bone metastases are a common cause of pain. Frequently the pain level varies according to the degree of mobility, and the addition of an anti-inflammatory agent such as aspirin or indomethacin to the drugs which the patient is already taking may help.

Pathological fractures should be splinted to reduce pain caused by movement of the body; inflatable splints are useful in this instance. Fracture boards placed under the mattress and a bedcradle to reduce the weight of bedclothes both help to reduce discomfort. A well covered hot-water bottle on the painful site may help, but care must be taken that the water is not boiling.

The use of a short-acting analgesic such as Entonox while carrying out procedures which are likely to cause pain, such as changing the patient's position or giving a bedpan, can be useful. (Entonox is a mixture of 50% nitrous oxide and 50% oxygen. Its administration is controlled by the patient who holds the delivery mask to his face himself – in this way he cannot get an over-dose since the mask will fall away as the inhaled gases take effect.)

Intractable vomiting

This can cause great misery and result in admission to hospital in an attempt to seek relief. The patient is often exhausted from the continual retching and vomiting, and becomes increasingly thirsty because of dehydration. If a cause of the vomiting is diagnosed then it may be possible to care for the patient at home. The district nurse should never overlook constipation as a cause of vomiting. The use of dexamethasone to treat raised intercranial pressure can give welcome remission. Intestinal obstruction, with its accompanying abdominal pain and nausea, can be helped, at least in the early stages, by a softening aperient combined with analgesics and anti-emetics. An antispasmodic such as lomotil may also be needed.

Anti-emetics such as prochlorperazine (Stemetil) are available as suppositories. If the patient has relatives capable of administering these suppositories then the district nurse can show them the procedure for insertion and then watch while they do this initially. Alternatively, she may have to visit herself for this purpose.

When the patient is no longer able to manage solid foods, nutrition is maintained by giving plenty of fluids, especially drinks such as Complan and Ensure. Gradually the need for these will diminish until during the last few days only frequent small drinks and crushed ice to suck are needed.

Sore mouth

Oral hygiene is important in the prevention of sore mouths and monilial infection and this should be explained to the patient and carers by the community nursing staff from the outset. Regular mouthwashes, using a solution such as Oraldene, after meals and after attacks of vomiting help to keep the mouth clean and free from food particles. Fungilin (amphotericin) lozenges can be sucked prophylactically three-hourly if monilial infection is a recurrent problem. Lipsalve or glycerine and borax are good for dry, cracked lips. Sucking acid fruit sweets or pineapple chunks stimulates the salivary glands producing saliva to moisten a dry mouth. Half an effervescent vitamin C tablet is useful for cleaning a coated tongue.

Constipation

Many dying patients suffer from constipation. Apart from mechanical systemic causes, this is because of lack of exercise, a diet low in roughage and the effect of the analgesic drugs. Aperients such as danthron (Dorbanex) need to be given routinely to most patients who are receiving regular opiate drugs. It is good nursing policy for the district nurse to carry out a rectal examination every three to four days on those patients known to suffer from constipation or who cannot be relied upon to give an accurate report of their bowel movements. If necessary a small enema or suppositories can then be given.

Anorexia

Anorexia is a common problem in malignant disease. The prescription of glucocorticosteroids by the GP will produce better appetite and a sense of well-being in many cases. The nurse can advise relatives how to deal with this problem. Usually smaller portions of attractively prepared food will be enjoyed, especially a favourite dish as opposed to traditional invalid foods. Alcohol before or with meals may help if the patient fancies it.

Dyspnoea

In the dying patient, attacks of dyspnoea can be extremely frightening and, if the cause is obstructive, may be difficult to relieve. The district nurse should advise relatives how to keep the patient propped up and supported with pillows either in bed or a chair. The window should be opened slightly for fresh air; psychologically this is important. The doctor may need to be contacted, as often the only relief from dyspnoea is sedation with opiates which lessen the intolerable sensation of asphyxia. If the patient is already taking oral diamorphine, this may have to be supplemented by intramuscular diamorphine at night when attacks tend to occur. Aminophylline suppositories occasionally help relieve the symptoms.

Cough

Continuous coughing can be very exhausting if the patient is weak, Simple Linctus BP is helpful and should be given frequently. Inhalations of warm, moist air from a steam kettle or a jug inhalation of Compound Tincture of Benzoin BPC (friar's balsam) often relieves a hacking cough. The nurse should supervise all inhalations. Even rubbing a 'sore chest' with Vick has a soothing and psychological effect. The patient *feels* something is being done. If the cough is productive then an expectorant can be prescribed during the day, with an antitussive agent at night.

Pressure sores

Prevention is better than cure and every effort must be made to prevent their occurrence. Pressure sores add greatly to a patient's discomfort and once they occur they are difficult to treat because they take so long to heal. The nurse must be aware of the possibility of their forming in a debilitated, thin and undernourished patient. The regular use of the 'Norton' pressure sore risk calculator (Table 6/1) will help her to highlight this risk and take measures to reduce it. The patient is assessed under five categories: physical condition, mental condition, activity, mobility and incontinent. A score is given for each category, 4 being good and 1 being poor. The score is totalled and if it is 14 or lower the patient is at risk of developing pressure sores and needs intensive nursing care to prevent their formation.

There are many predisposing factors but the main agents in pressure sore formation are continuous direct pressure and shearing forces. Thus when planning care for the terminally ill patient the district nurse should bear in mind the physiological

Table 6/1 The 'Norton' pressure sore risk calculator

A	B	C	D	E
Physical condition	Mental condition	Activity	Mobility	Incontinent
4 Good	4 Alert	4 Ambulant	4 Full	4 Not
3 Fair	3 Apathetic	3 Walk/help	3 Slightly limited	3 Occasion-ally
2 Poor	2 Confused	2 Chairbound	2 Very limited	2 Usually/ urine
1 Very bad	1 Stuporous	1 Bedfast	1 Immobile	1 Doubly

facts relevant to the formation of pressure sores and assess how 'at risk' he is of developing such sores. The next step is to take action to prevent this and to educate the caring relatives to continue this prevention throughout the 24 hours.

Advice on the prevention of pressure sores

- Encourage the patient to remain mobile for as long as possible, even if this only means getting up to go to the toilet.
- Once in bed encourage him to change his position from time to time. If necessary help him to turn from side to side every two hours.
- Regularly inspect those areas subject to pressure to detect early any signs of soreness. Areas at risk include the shoulders, elbows, sacral region and buttocks, trochanters, knees and heels. The lobes of the ears and the base of the skull should be watched also.
- Relieve pressure on these areas by using rings, pads or carefully placed pillows. Other useful aids include sheepskins and alternating pressure mattresses.
- Keep the skin clean and dry. If the patient is incontinent, wash his hips and buttocks each time the sheets are changed and dry the skin well before applying a protective barrier cream. Any vigorous rubbing of existing 'paper thin' skin is contra-indicated.
- The use of a cream such as Vasogen or Thovaline applied to buttocks, heels and other bony prominences helps to keep dry skin supple and so prevent cracks from developing.
- Ensure that the bottom sheet is kept smooth and free from crumbs.
- When lifting the patient ensure that he is lifted clear of the bed so that delicate skin is not damaged by friction caused by rubbing against the bottom sheet.
- Use a footboard or pillows wrapped in a drawsheet to prevent him from slipping down the bed and so putting shearing forces into play.
- If, in spite of all these preventive measures, sores do occur, treat them as surgical wounds.
- Do not forget that patients can become sore when two skin surfaces are rubbing together especially if moisture is also present in the form of sweat or urine. Heavy pendulous breasts can become red and sore underneath in this way.

Many treatments are used by district nurses for pressure sores, but the important principle is the relief of pressure. Any slough should be removed before the wound is packed with gauze soaked in a solution which aids healing. Oxygen and ultraviolet light are sometimes used to speed up the process of healing. Ample protein and vitamins should be included in the patient's diet.

Insomnia

Often sleep does not come easily to the dying patient. In this case nursing care includes making sure the patient does not want to go to the lavatory, is not in pain, is quite comfortable in bed, has taken a hot milky drink (possibly laced with alcohol) and has a covered hot-water bottle placed on any aching area of his body. If these simple measures fail, then the district nurse should ask the GP to prescribe a sedative such as temazepam which induces a more normal sleep, and has a short half life. Some patients settle better after taking dichloralphenazone (Welldorm) or chlormethiazole (Heminevrin).

Fungating tumours

A fungating carcinoma of the breast is a most distressing condition, and the sight and smell can be quite upsetting. The patient needs a great deal of reassurance, and the nurse should not show any signs of distaste because this would make the patient even more embarrassed and self-conscious. In most cases, local applications are the only possible means of continual treatment. Regular cleaning of the area is extremely important. In such cases the district nurse visits daily, sometimes twice daily, to re-dress the lesion. Various cleansing agents can be used such as eusol and paraffin (one part in four); equal volumes of eusol and water; 4% povidone-iodine (Betadine skin cleanser). Yogurt is a popular application for fungating tumours. It is easier for the nurse to wear sterile disposable gloves for this procedure because she can clean this type of wound more gently by using her hands instead of forceps. A local antibiotic such as Polybactrin spray can then be used to combat local sepsis. Alternative dressings include impregnated tulle gras such as Sofra-Tulle and Fucidin Intertulle. A non-adhesive dressing such as Melolin is applied over the tulle gras with a cotton-wool pad placed on top and taped or bandaged into position. If there is a foul odour the nurse can use special dressings containing charcoal, which will absorb the smell, and a course of systemic antibiotics may help to reduce sepsis with its associated offensive discharge. Air purifiers may be obtained on loan. The district nurse should keep the GP informed about the patient's condition and the progressive nature of the fungating lesion.

Incontinence

Symptoms of frequency and incontinence are often found in patients with advanced malignant disease. Catheterisation should be considered if the incontinence cannot be controlled by treatment of urinary tract infections or the use of anticholinergic drugs to increase the bladder's capacity.

The risks associated with long-term catheterisation do not apply to this category of patient, as the main consideration is to keep him as comfortable as possible and also to abide by his wishes.

Depression

Where the patient is aware of his condition, depression is a natural consequence. This is partly ascribed to fear of the unknown mixed with sorrow at the thought of leaving behind family, friends and familiar surroundings. In the patient who is unaware of his diagnosis, depression can be due to weariness and uncertainty after a protracted illness which shows no signs of abating.

At this stage the patient's attitudes to dying may be examined more closely; they will largely depend on the course of the disease, personal experiences and environmental influences. Various fears are common:

Being alone: He may refuse sedation or analgesics or sleeping drugs; he may sleep in the day and be awake and demanding at night. Some people who know their prognosis do not want their family to witness their death as they do not want them to be upset but would rather they remembered them as they were when fit and well.

Powerlessness: The patient might prefer a sudden death but on the other hand he might wish to live as long as possible with everything done to prolong his life. He may wish to make his own decisions about where he should die. Hospital admission may be refused or he may not adhere to treatment regimes.

Dependence: Independence is highly valued. The patient may worry about coping with personal hygiene, his food and his toilet requirements. In fact he may become rebellious or be angry and frustrated at his weakness.

We are all unique individuals who have our own ways of reacting to the knowledge of advancing death. Denying death is a coping strategy for one is then manufacturing hopes for the future. The patient may regress to simpler times and this may be expressed in his interests and daily activities. Anger may be intense or mild. 'Why?' questions abound. Often a person's reaction to approaching death depends upon his age. The elderly are often more occupied with their physical disabilities than with any emotional turmoil of dying. They are more trusting of what the doctor has told them; the young demand to know.

The district nurse's intervention should allow her to support coping behaviours, to facilitate the development of coping strategies, to modify maladaptive behaviours, to foster patient growth and awareness during the dying process and to promote the quality of living until the time of death.

Other problems

Various aspects have to be considered when assessing the suitability of the home for nursing a terminally ill patient. Although the home itself may not be ideal, yet, in spite of inconvenience and discomfort, it can still be the best place in which to die. The need for familiar and well-loved surroundings far outweighs anything which a hospital can offer. In many cases, not only is it best for the patient, but it is better for the family who need the opportunity to express their love before it is too late. This is the ideal situation, but unfortunately not every dying patient has relatives who are willing or fit enough to care for them with the heavy nursing involved. All too frequently it happens that an elderly spouse has to care for the other partner without any family support and often in completely unsuitable conditions. It is the sheer physical exhaustion of the caring relative which usually necessitates the hospital admission of the patient. Weekends and nights can be a special anxiety, as in many areas there is not a full 24-hour NHS coverage for patients at home. Once the medical centre or surgery has closed for the night or weekend, the telephone number is either referred to another GP or a central agency. This means the patient and his family are cut off from their own doctor, who knows all about them, unless it happens to be his turn 'on call' for the practice. The district nurse may be the only regular visitor, but she is there for relatively short periods during the daytime. Some areas do have a comprehensive 24-hour nursing coverage; others have a 'twilight nursing service'; while some have an 'on-call' rota for their daytime district nurses to carry out essential late evening duties such as injections of analgesics or night sedations. Most areas have arrangements for night nurses to be provided for the terminally ill cancer patient on a short-term basis, usually one or two nights a week, funded by the Marie Curie Memorial Foundation. More health authorities are now employing nursing auxiliaries to sit with seriously ill patients during the night. The British Red Cross Society and St John Ambulance Brigade can sometimes help by finding volunteer members who are willing to sit with a dying patient to allow the family to have some rest. If no help is available the resulting broken nights often make home care by the family impossible and result in the patient's admission to hospital.

Financial aspects of care

When a patient is admitted to hospital the full cost of his care is borne by the National Health Service and all he loses is part of his pension or allowances. At home his family shoulders a considerable financial burden; he needs special foods, extra heating and repeated prescriptions for drugs and dressings which, if he is under pensionable age, can be very expensive. Time off work because of illness or caring for a sick person can result in a loss of earnings and cause financial hardship. A family is not eligible for Attendance Allowance if the illness is of less than six months' duration. Supplementary grants are often inadequate but the district nurse should remember that financial help is available from some charitable organisations and if necessary these should be approached with the permission of patient or family.

Laundry

Services, such as an incontinent laundry service and the collection of offensive contaminated dressings and pads, vary from district to district. Where the service is available the district nurse can request collection on behalf of her patient. Even so, the sheer volume of clean laundry required to keep the patient clean and happy is an extra strain on those caring for the patient, and as a consequence can lead to his admission to hospital so that they may be given a rest.

DEATH

When the patient's respiration becomes deep and stertorous, and the periods of apnoea increase, the district nurse, if present, should gently tell the family that death is approaching. If at all possible she should arrange for someone to remain with them at this time. However, if prevented from doing so because of work commitments, she should quietly tell one of the family what to do when the patient stops breathing. First, they should inform the doctor; while waiting for him they should lay the patient flat in bed with a small pillow under the head, close the eyes if open and put a small pillow under the chin to support it.

When the doctor calls, he will sign the death certificate, advise the family how to register the death and how to contact an undertaker. Grieving relatives do not think clearly at this time, so the nurse may need to reinforce the doctor's instructions. It often helps to write down as much information as possible.

Generally in the community, Last Offices are carried out by the undertaker. The district nurse, if present at the time of death, will lay the dead person flat on the bed, ensuring that the dentures (if any) are in place and that the eyes are closed, with a piece of damp gauze or cotton wool over each eye to keep the lids in place. She will remove any tubes, catheters or intravenous infusions before covering the body with a sheet.

After the patient has died, the speedy removal of equipment and disposal of unused drugs should be undertaken. Each district has its own policy which should be adhered to by the district nurse. If the house is connected to the main drainage the correct course is to flush Controlled Drugs down the lavatory and ask a relative to witness this. Burning is another means of disposing of such drugs.

Bereavement

Although the district nurse's duty to her patient ends with his death, she still has to consider the welfare of the family left behind. Time spent in listening to expressions of grief or in telling stories of years gone by can be of great value in helping the family to accept their loss and start off on the path to normal living again. Having shared the role of caring with them, the district nurse becomes a trusted family friend; someone with whom they can discuss their problems, and who can advise them on how to cope with living again after their loss.

Many district nurses visit 10 to 14 days after the patient's death when the funeral is over; by this time relatives may have returned to their respective homes leaving the close family on their own, often only too happy to have a listener. At this time some idea can be gained as to the extent of family support; the financial situation; the reaction of any children to the death; the bereaved's own feelings and whether any help is needed. The nurse often makes a casual visit several months later to satisfy herself that all is well and that no further help is needed. If she is concerned about the reactions of the bereaved person then obviously she will visit more frequently and if necessary inform the GP of her concern.

HELPFUL ORGANISATIONS

Macmillan Nurses

Douglas Macmillan founded the National Society for Cancer Relief (NSCR) in 1911 with the aim of disseminating information on the prevention and relief of cancer. It registered as a benevolent society in 1924 and then concentrated on giving financial aid to cancer patients. In the early 1970s, when hospice care was developing, the NSCR took the initiative to make such care more widely available. Grants were given; then, working with the NHS, it created its own programme of building Macmillan Continuing Care Homes. In 1979 a new emphasis was given to extending cancer care into the community. Macmillan domiciliary care services were initially given to certain hospices. In 1980 a huge investment of £2½ million (over 3 years) enabled Macmillan nursing teams to be established, to work with the Primary Health Care Teams in caring for cancer patients in their own homes.

Macmillan nurses are experienced district nurses or health visitors who have undertaken the English National Board Course 930 in 'Care of the Dying Patient and his Family'. They use their special knowledge to advise on the relief of pain and other distressing symptoms and give emotional support to the whole family.

The Marie Curie Memorial Foundation

The Marie Curie Memorial Foundation was established in 1948 and is an independent voluntary organisation. It provides a comprehensive service for cancer patients, including:

1. The provision of 11 residential homes for patients with cancer throughout the UK.
2. The provision of nursing and other assistance for cancer patients being cared for at home. (The cost of providing night nurses is usually shared with the NHS and the community nurse managers organise the scheme locally.)
3. The provision of general information, advice and counselling on cancer for the general public.
4. The funding of research relating to cancer.

BIBLIOGRAPHY

Charles-Edwards, A. (1983). *The Nursing Care of the Dying Patient.* Beaconsfield Publishers, Beaconsfield.

Copperman, H. (1983). *Dying at Home.* J. Wiley and Sons, Chichester.

Corr, C.A. and Corr, D.M. (jt eds) (1983). *Hospice Care: Principles and Practice.* Faber and Faber, London; Springer Publishing Company, Inc, New York.

Dealing with Death and Dying. A Nursing Skillbook. (1976). Ravenswood Publications, Beckenham.

Hinton, J. (1971). *Dying.* Penguin Books, Harmondsworth.

Kubler-Ross, E. (1970). *Death and Dying.* Tavistock Publications, London.

Parkes, C.M. (1975). *Bereavement: Studies of Grief in Adult Life.* Penguin Books, Harmondsworth.

Chapter Seven

THE STROKE PATIENT

Not all stroke patients are admitted to hospital. Many are cared for at home by their families, supported by regular visits from the district nurse. Those who do go into hospital are usually referred back to the care of the district nurse on discharge. She is the person most concerned with his nursing care and shares his rehabilitation with the physiotherapist, occupational therapist and speech therapist. The district nurse has several roles to play when it comes to caring for the stroke patient at home. She is primarily responsible for his nursing care until he achieves independence. She provides psychological support and encouragement to both the patient and his family and is their teacher and demonstrator. He needs to know what he can do to help himself and they need to know how to nurse and care for him. It is extremely important that the district nurse should liaise closely with the physiotherapist so that she can reinforce any instructions given to the patient and his family. Ideally she should attend a physiotherapy session with her patient to facilitate continuity of care and ensure that she follows local practice in the supervising of any movements and exercises.

THE DISTRICT NURSE'S FIRST VISIT

At the nurse's first visit, she assesses the domestic situation as well as the physical and mental state of the patient. The amount of help available to care for the patient is important because an elderly spouse cannot be expected to cope alone with a severely handicapped or unconscious patient. If younger relatives are able to help then a plan of nursing care can be discussed and the district nurse can show them how to care for their sick relative. Often the first few nights can be difficult and so she must enquire if two people can stay overnight until the patient improves.

It is important to spend time talking to the family, who are probably shocked by this crisis and need to be able to ask questions and gain practical advice and help.

THE UNCONSCIOUS PATIENT

If the patient is unconscious when the nurse visits, she must see that the dentures are removed and that he is nursed on his side. This allows the tongue to fall forward ensuring a clear airway. One of the family should be involved in helping the district nurse to position and care for the patient at this stage. The importance of this positioning and the need for two-hourly turning to relieve pressure on the bony prominences and prevent pressure sores should be emphasised by the district nurse at this time. While showing the family how to turn and wash the patient she will protect the mattress with a plastic drawsheet and place incontinence pads under the patient's buttocks. Catheterisation is avoided if possible at this early stage, but if it becomes necessary then the catheter should be removed as soon as possible when the patient recovers.

It may be that when the nurse arrives the patient is still fully clothed because the advent of the stroke was recent and the family have been too scared to touch him or worried about hurting him. In this case she will have to ask for help to undress the patient and will give advice on how best to handle and move him while he is being undressed. She must not forget that family members may well be embarrassed initially at having to help with such intimate tasks. Her instructions on how to care for the patient at this time often help to overcome this temporary embarrassment.

The district nurse should show the relatives how to clean the patient's mouth to prevent it from becoming dry and infected. Cotton Buds or cotton wool wrapped around an orange stick or teaspoon handle, dipped in a solution of bicarbonate of soda (one teaspoon to a glass of water) helps to dissolve mucus and clean the mouth. The lips should be moistened with glycerine or Lipsalve to prevent cracking.

Eye care is also very important if the patient is unconscious and unable to blink. Relatives should be shown how to wipe the eyes with a cotton-wool swab moistened with normal saline (one teaspoon salt to a pint of water). A drop of liquid paraffin should be instilled to moisten the surface of the eye.

If the patient remains unconscious for more than 24 hours, a decision must be made regarding the institution of nasogastric feeding to maintain nutrition and prevent dehydration. This intensive nursing care may be too arduous for the family and hospital admission may be requested. If the patient continues to be cared for at home the district nurse may visit several times a day to assist in the caring process and to evaluate progress. On her first visit she will also assess what equipment is needed to help in providing nursing care and preventing complications. The loan of a ripple bed or other mattress designed to relieve pressure may be requested by the nurse. A bedcradle can be obtained so as to prevent the weight of the bedclothes pressing on the legs and feet and so causing contractures or footdrop. Incontinence pads and sheets may need to be supplied together with a waterproof cream to protect the buttocks from the effects of continual contact with acid urine. Relatives should be reminded about the importance of regularly changing wet pads and washing and drying the patient's buttocks and applying the cream.

CONTINUING CARE

Much will depend upon the patient's progress and the severity of the initial stroke. If the stroke has been less severe then the patient may be sat out of bed for a short while and his family can be shown how to help him out of bed into a chair, or on to a commode. The community physiotherapist and occupational therapist should be involved with the stroke patient as soon as possible. They will individually and/or jointly assess the patient's needs for rehabilitation and show the district nurse and relatives how they can help in the rehabilitation process. Useful books about rehabilitation are listed on page 81 but it is important for the nurse to follow the methods of rehabilitation practised locally.

Those aspects of rehabilitation which the district nurse should be teaching the patient and his family in conjunction with her physiotherapy and occupational therapy colleagues include:

positioning in lying in bed
good sitting posture and the need for a firm table in front of the
    patient who is in a chair for safety
how to move from side to side in bed
how to reach sitting from lying
how to transfer from the bed to a chair and back again.

In addition other aspects of daily activities will need to be considered.

Eating and drinking

Swallowing is often a problem for the stroke patient, so much so that there is a danger that he could become dehydrated from inadequate fluid intake. There is also a danger of inhalation pneumonia if the patient drinks while lying so it is important that the district nurse teaches relatives how to position the patient upright in a good sitting posture before helping him to have a drink. She must be aware of how upsetting and degrading these problems with eating and drinking are for the patient and his family. Because of a loss of facial nerve function on the affected side the patient may not be aware that his lips are open and is unable to feel the presence of saliva, a spoon or cup. Food may collect in a flaccid pouch in the affected cheek and so oral hygiene following a meal is another important aspect of care which the district nurse must teach. She should also teach how to assist swallowing by a standard drill:

1. Teeth together
2. Lips together
3. When ready to swallow hold the breath (if possible after an inspiration)
4. Swallow
5. Continue breathing!

The help of a dental surgeon at this stage can be useful because dentures can be modified and special appliances provided to help rehabilitation. Once it is established that the patient is able to swallow fluids the district nurse should advise that he should be given a little and often as there is still a danger of dehydration. He should be offered suitably well-flavoured foods and good suggestions for starters are ice cream, stewed apple and tinned peaches.

Elimination

There is a danger that because of his immobility the patient could become constipated and eventually suffer from incontinence of faeces due to impaction. The district nurse should be aware of this and take steps to prevent it. She should advise the relatives about providing a well-balanced diet containing cereal, vegetable roughage and plenty of fluids. Bran sprinkled on cereals or stews is a useful idea. If constipation is already a problem the district nurse may need to give a simple enema or suppository.

Most stroke patients are incontinent initially but as soon as he is able and fit enough he should be helped out on to a commode at regular intervals in an attempt to re-establish reflex emptying. The dysphasic patient has extra problems in that he is unable to indicate when he wishes to use the toilet, so the assistance of the speech therapist can be invaluable. Some patients never regain bladder control, and some prefer catheterisation as opposed to continually having to put up with wearing wet pads and protective pants. The district nurse should discuss the alternatives with the patient and his family and allow him the opportunity to try them out.

As the patient progresses and gets up for a longer time each day he should be encouraged to do more for himself. There is a danger that relatives will tend to over-protect him and the nurse must explain that they are not really helping him by doing this.

Dressing

If he attends occupational therapy and physiotherapy sessions, the patient will receive training in how to dress himself. If he is at home it is the district nurse (or community occupational therapist) who will teach the patient and relatives how to manage with dressing and undressing. It is always so much easier, and quicker, to be kind and do things for the stroke patient but it is more beneficial to allow him to struggle for a while and give only spoken help. Initially, it is easier to practise dressing while still on the bed. As balance improves he can sit on the side of the bed with his feet supported; he may need support to stand and pull up underclothes and trousers. (See pages 81, 118 and 190 for helpful handbooks.)

Standing and walking

Walking practice should be taught and supervised initially by a physiotherapist who can then teach the district nurse the most effective way of reinforcing the instructions. It cannot be over-emphasised that the correct gait training in the early stages is vital to re-establishing a successful pattern of walking. Close liaison with therapists is so important for the district nurse who must be aware of the principles behind any stroke rehabilitation so that, in the event of there not being a physiotherapist available in her area, she can efficiently mobilise the patient in his own home and demonstrate to relatives how best they can help.

Ascending and descending stairs

Unless the patient lives in a bungalow or ground floor flat, or is likely to be rehoused, he will need to learn how to manage stairs. The community occupational therapist should be consulted about the provision of extra handrails; if the stair treads are too high it may be necessary to provide half-steps and the occupational therapist should be able to advise. In helping patients to manage to negotiate stairs, it is better if the helper descends in front of the patient, facing him, as he comes down the stairs, and stays behind him as he ascends.

Bathing

Some patients may not have a bathroom and so the nurse will wash the parts of the body which the patient cannot reach. If the bathroom is suitable, the district nurse can ask the occupational therapist to visit with her to assess what aids may be required. Rails can be fitted and mats, bath boards and bath seats provided. Often, once the patient has achieved a degree of independence, the only reason for the district nurse to visit is to help with bathing. One method is described:

The patient sits on a chair in the bathroom to undress. This chair is placed so that his strong side is next to the bath. The bath board is fixed across the bath next to the patient and the bath seat is wedged into the bath farther down from the board. The patient is then helped to transfer from the chair to sit on the bath board facing away from the bath. He is asked to wriggle back on the board, and then, holding the side of the bath, he places his good leg into the bath as the nurse helps the weak leg. As he becomes more adept he may be able to tuck his stronger leg under the weaker one and manage to get both legs into the bath unaided. Holding the bath edge with his strong hand and supported by the nurse on his weak side he then slides down on to the bath seat. (If the bath is up against the wall, a holding rail will need to be fixed.)

The bath should be emptied before any attempt is made to help the patient out. Then, the patient holds the bath edge (or rail) with his strong hand, bends the knee of his strong leg, while the nurse, supporting him under his weak axilla, asks him to push himself straight up and on to the board. He then moves towards the edge of the bath and, with the nurse lifting his weak leg out of the bath, the patient lifts his strong leg out turning at the same time to sit facing outwards. He may prefer to dry himself in this position or he may prefer to do so in his chair, in which case a large towel should be draped over the whole chair so that he can be wrapped in it.

Aphasia and speech therapy

The extreme frustration of having something to say and being unable to make anyone understand can be distressing and may cause severe depression. The nurse and family should not try to rush the patient, but should encourage him to express himself in other ways. This might be the use of hand gestures, or the repeating of a word, as soon as she knows what it is the patient wants to say. Sentences should be short and simple. Speech therapy is important but may be difficult to arrange in some areas. Nurses, relatives and friends must, therefore, help a great deal with this aspect of rehabilitation.

Useful advice on how to help an aphasic patient includes the following:

Always try the written word if the spoken word is not successful, as the patient may be deaf as well as aphasic

Speak slowly and distinctly and if necessary point to articles or pictures in order to make yourself understood

The fewest possible words should be used

Make use of hand gestures

Get the patient's attention by standing in his line of vision

A word and picture chart (published by the Chest, Heart and Stroke Association) can be used to communicate basic needs such as 'drink', 'book' and 'lavatory'.

Relief for the family

When a district nurse visits any patient she must be concerned not only about his health and welfare, but also that the strain of caring does not become too great for the relatives. For the stroke patient attendance at a (geriatric) day hospital not only allows for intensive physiotherapy and occupational therapy on several days a week but also means that the family can have a break from caring and some time to themselves. Attendance at a day hospital is usually for a limited time during which active rehabilitation takes place. Once the patient is discharged from their care he may be able to attend a day centre or stroke club once or twice a week. This will provide him with social contact and give some respite to relatives. It also enables the patient to realise that he is not alone in being disabled in this way.

If the patient is severely handicapped and is a strain on those caring for him, the district nurse may discuss with the family, the GP and possibly the social worker the referral of the patient for shared care or holiday admissions.

The role of the district nurse in caring for a patient who has had a stroke is concerned primarily with providing the basic nursing care necessary to ensure patient comfort and prevent the onset of complications. Once the critical stage is over, she is concerned with the rehabilitative aspects of care and becomes adviser and teacher to both patient and relatives.

Some district nurses are involved in the preventive aspects of cerebrovascular disease by running hypertension screening clinics. If a raised blood pressure is discovered early enough in relatively young people and treated at this stage, it may prevent the development of widespread cerebrovascular disease later.

Caring for and rehabilitating the stroke patient involves a team which includes the patient, his family, the general practitioner, the district nurses, the therapists and voluntary workers. The district nurse is usually the person most intimately involved in the care and management and is often the co-ordinator of this care.

BIBLIOGRAPHY

Bobath, B. (1978). *Adult Hemiplegia: Evaluation and Treatment*, 2nd *edition*. William Heinemann Medical Books Ltd, London.

Downie, P. A. and Kennedy, P. (1981). *Lifting, Handling and Helping Patients*. Faber and Faber, London.

Eaton Griffith, V. (1970). *A Stroke in the Family*. Wildwood House Ltd, London.

Hawker, M. (1978). *Return to Mobility: Exercises for the Stroke Patient*. Chest, Heart and Stroke Association, London.

Johnstone, M. (1976). *The Stroke Patient: Principles of Rehabilitation*. Churchill Livingstone, Edinburgh.

Jay, P. (1985). *Help Yourselves: A Handbook for Hemiplegics and Their Families*, 4th edition. Ian Henry Publications, Hornchurch.

Lubbock, G. (ed) (1983). *Stroke Care: An Interdisciplinary Approach.* Faber and Faber, London.

Chapter Eight

CARING FOR THE ELDERLY AT HOME

Over a million elderly people are treated annually by district nurses – this is well over half of the district nurse's workload. An increasing number of elderly in the community means more people with disability and chronic degenerative diseases, yet only 9 per cent of trained nurses work in the community.

PLANNING CARE FOR THE ELDERLY AT HOME

The main aim when a district nurse visits the home of an elderly person for the first time is the achievement of an improved state of health, independence and comfort. She may direct her help towards the prevention or delay of a potentially disabling condition, or towards the detection of illness. This initial visit is to assess the needs of the patient and to plan his care (see Chapter 2). It also serves as a time to establish mutual understanding.

Having completed her assessment, and before leaving the house, the district nurse should discuss with the patient, and any family present at the time, the care that is needed and what steps she would like to take. She should indicate when she will call again. She will also explain that she will contact the various agencies whose help is needed.

Effects of housing on the health of the individual

The health of an elderly person living in a slum area is generally inferior to one living in good housing conditions. The majority of poor houses are damp because of defective roofing or guttering, or there may be rising damp due to lack of a damp-proof course. Damp exacerbates rheumatic problems, aggravates chronic bronchitis, and has a depressing effect on the occupant. One finds that it is the elderly person who suffers mostly from bad housing.

In a modern house, a downstairs room can be turned into a temporary bedroom in which the patient can be nursed. In a slum dwelling with an outside lavatory, continence is not helped!

Old people need to live in warm, comfortable, well-lit accommodation, if possible on one level. Even today the district nurse visiting a rural area finds her patient living in an old, damp cottage without sanitation and sometimes without a piped water supply. Here hot water and baths are rare and cooking is often done on a coal range or oil-burning stove. To be ill in such conditions is not conducive to a quick recovery, although in country areas there is often great community spirit and help is more readily given. In big cities life can be lonely for the elderly, but social services are in better supply. Town houses belonging to elderly people are often dark, cold, cluttered up with heavy furniture, loose mats, awkward steps and primitive kitchen and toilet arrangements. In such conditions the risk of home accidents is increased.

Bearing in mind that her aim is to help and encourage independence wherever possible, the district nurse must consider the effect the patient's home conditions are having on his health.

(a) Is the accommodation suitable for the patient to remain where he is, given adequate support?
(b) What are his own feelings? The nurse must discuss possibilities with the patient and plan her course of action with his approval.
(c) The social worker must be consulted and her opinion sought when considering housing grants, sheltered housing or residential accommodation.
(d) Is a 'granny flat' the answer for those with sufficient financial resources?

Financial assistance for the elderly

Income maintenance for the elderly can come from the following sources:

Social security benefits including

(a) Retirement pensions – available to all pensioners
(b) Graduated pensions – added in respect of any graduated contributions paid between 1961 and 1975 (when these ceased)
(c) An addition of 25p a week to all pensioners aged 80 or over
(d) Supplementary pensions and rent and rate rebates

Private occupational pension schemes
Benevolent funds and charitable trusts
Assurance schemes
Attendance allowance

For elderly people to remain in the community, they not only need an adequate income, but also suitable housing. Many lack the necessary knowledge for obtaining their entitlements. Although the district nurse has been asked to visit her elderly patient because he is in need of nursing care, she cannot ignore his other needs which may be slowing down his physical recovery.

NUTRITIONAL PROBLEMS
OF THE ELDERLY

Older citizens may know very little about food values and vitamins, and their eating habits become very limited. Elderly people living alone tend to lose interest in preparing meals for themselves; their loneliness leads to boredom, depression, apathy and subsequent self-neglect.

The distance to the shops is another factor in the development of undernutrition. A frail elderly person may find it difficult to walk far to do shopping and carry it all home. In a busy street it is an ordeal for a disabled pensioner to cross to the other side to get to the butcher or greengrocer, so he does not do so and thus restricts his diet. As disablement progresses, switching on the gas or electricity becomes a problem, as can the lifting of a heavy saucepan or kettle. All this effort, together with the increasing cost of meat and vegetables, result in many elderly people resorting to the cheaper convenience, carbohydrate foods which are easier to obtain and prepare.

The district nurse will realise that she cannot immediately change the dietary routine of perhaps a lifetime. She will first have to build up a relationship with her patient, gain his trust and discover his regular diet. Explanations of why certain items should be included are essential in order to persuade him to change to a more nutritious way of eating. It helps if the cheapest forms of nourishing food are the ones recommended.

It should not be forgotten that elderly patients may have relatives or neighbours willing to do shopping or possibly cook for them, but that they may be unaware that the person is having difficulty in coping and is too proud to ask for help. Other alternatives include:

Meals on wheels

This service is of great assistance to those who are too old and frail to cook and cater for themselves. Unfortunately it is not available seven days a week and services are sometimes limited by the locality in rural areas. A small charge is made for this hot two-course meal but it is subsidised by the local authority who also usually provide help with equipment and cooking facilities. In many areas, the actual service is run by the Women's Royal Voluntary Service (WRVS) whose members deliver the meals which have been prepared in a central kitchen. More use is being made of pre-cooked meals in foil containers which only need heating.

Attendance at luncheon clubs

These clubs are of value for the elderly person who is neglecting his dietary needs because he lives alone and has become apathetic and depressed with his solitary existence. Attendance at such a club would help him physically and improve his mental outlook.

Home helps

Home helps are the mainstay of elderly people who wish to remain in their own homes and yet are too frail to cope with all that this entails. The home help service is run by the local authority through its social services department, and as it is financed through the local rates, the extent of the service varies from one authority to another. Elderly people are usually charged on a sliding scale but the service may be provided free to those relying solely on their pension and who have high rents and other expenses.

Home helps may be required to do housework, shopping, collecting the pension, cleaning windows and, if necessary, cooking a meal on those days when the meals on wheels scheme does not function.

Good neighbour schemes

Many local authorities finance these schemes. They are often arranged through the home help supervisor, who visits the elderly person to discuss his needs and then makes enquiries locally to see if there is a neighbour (often a housewife) who could visit regularly to help with simple but necessary tasks beyond his capabilities.

Day centres

Day centres may be run by the local authority and some are financed by charities. They offer more than luncheon clubs as the elderly person can spend the whole day at the centre, have a hot mid-day meal, and participate in the social activities provided.

Volunteers

The district nurse often meets an elderly person whose needs are not catered for by the statutory services and it is then that she contacts a member of one of the local voluntary organisations concerned with the welfare of elderly people. Age Concern is one of the most widely known organisations concerned with the care of the elderly.

HEALTH AUTHORITY SERVICES FOR THE ELDERLY

As the number of elderly persons living in the community continues to increase, so the skills of the district nurse should be utilised to the full. In many areas, nursing auxiliaries are employed to carry out straightforward tasks such as bathing elderly patients, getting them out of bed, dressing them and washing their hair as necessary. The trained nurse carries out any skilled nursing procedures and visits all patients to assess their needs and monitor their progress. She liaises with all who are concerned with the patient's welfare.

The health visitor

While the district nurse is referred to the home of an elderly person for a specific purpose, the health visitor has to seek out those elderly members of the community in need and put them in touch with the appropriate services. Health visitors who are attached to general practice teams have the vital function of visiting those patients who are most vulnerable. In some areas there are health visitors who specialise in visiting the elderly and are attached to a department of geriatric medicine. They form a link between hospital and the patient's home, carrying out follow-up visits to ensure that all is satisfactory, and that no relapse is occurring, reporting to the hospital doctors and GP on the patient's progress and condition. It is important that district nurses and health visitors should work *together* in caring for the elderly patient and avoid overlapping.

The general practitioner

Old people make more calls on the time of the GP than the younger generations, and this is partly because their needs are often half social and half medical. For this reason, close liaison with the district nurse and health visitor is essential when planning care for the elderly sick. The amount of time devoted to routine visiting of elderly patients varies from practice to practice. Some doctors try to visit every three months, others may arrange a yearly check visit, and still others may only visit when requested. Since few elderly patients report symptoms at the time when they might be cured, this latter policy is the least desirable, unless there is a geriatric screening scheme being carried out.

Geriatric day hospitals

Day hospitals are part of the local department of geriatric medicine and consequently the patients are under the direct care of the consultant geriatrician. The day hospital has various functions:

(a) To continue treatment begun elsewhere, for example, dressings, injections, physiotherapy or occupational therapy.
(b) To maintain treatment of patients recently discharged from the wards who are not yet fully independent.
(c) To prevent unnecessary admissions and readmissions.
(d) To provide rehabilitation for the disabled.
(e) To allow earlier discharge from geriatric wards.
(f) To allow a thorough investigation of a patient's condition and to treat accordingly.
(g) To evaluate treatment and medication.

Geriatric day hospitals are run on a Monday to Friday basis and between 15 and 40 patients may attend daily, depending on the facilities and space available. Most patients attend two or three times a week, and it is on the other days that the district nurse often plays her part in the treatment and rehabilitation of a day hospital patient. Close liaison is therefore essential to ensure continuity of care.

The remainder of this chapter deals with some of the health problems that the district nurse may discover when caring for elderly patients. She will find that they often suffer from more than one condition at a time because degeneration, infection or failure of one or more systems of the body has a widespread effect.

DEAFNESS

Deafness is a barrier to communication and is a problem among the older age-groups because they lose the high-pitched notes and when in a crowd they cannot separate one particular sound. The district nurse should try to discover how long the patient has had a hearing problem and whether this has been investigated. Figure 8/1 indicates possible courses of action.

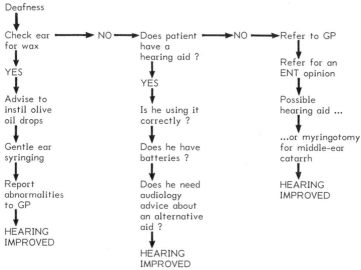

Fig. 8/1 Possible course(s) of action when deafness is present

VISUAL PROBLEMS

Most people as they get older are affected in varying degrees by presbyopia (difficulty in focusing on near objects). This is due to loss of elasticity of the lens capsule, and from middle age onward many people require reading glasses. As they grow older and less mobile, visits to the optician become difficult and expensive for the patient, and many people continue to use the same spectacles for many years. Their ability to read or do fine work declines and life consequently becomes tedious.

Some old people have to use magnifying glasses or special print magnifiers in order to read. These may be obtained from an optician, although in certain cases a prescription from a consultant ophthalmologist is needed. Libraries have a selection of large-print books, and usually a neighbour or home help will change the patient's books if he is unable to visit the library.

Cataract

Lens opacities or cataracts may be of slow onset and are often attributed to the gradual drop in vision that occurs with ageing. Once formed, senile cataracts can be dealt with by surgery. For an elderly person living alone the operation may be carried out sooner than in the case of someone living with his family. The former is likely to be kept in hospital longer than the latter. When discharged, he should be able to manage on his own with the supporting services visiting daily. This is important as his vision is considerably reduced and glasses are not prescribed until the surgeon sees him about six weeks postoperatively and refraction is carried out. The district nurse will visit to supervise the instillation of any eye drops prescribed by the surgeon and hopefully to educate a relative or the patient himself in the technique of instilling these essential drops, if this has not been done before he left hospital.

Glaucoma

One of the usual treatments of chronic, simple, open-angle glaucoma is the use of pilocarpine drops which, if prescribed in the early stages, may delay the progression of the condition. Again the district nurse must teach either a relative or friend how to instil these drops if the patient cannot manage for himself. Any gastro-intestinal side-effects such as nausea, vomiting, pain or abdominal cramps should be reported to the doctor.

Eventually, despite treatment, some patients lose their sight. If this seems likely, the patient should be encouraged to remain independent for as long as possible. He must concentrate on the use of his other senses, namely touch and hearing, and the use of a Zimmer frame (rather than a white stick) helps to prevent an elderly person tripping over objects in his path. The furniture should be left in accustomed places for the patient to hold on to, and any obvious obstacles removed.

TEETH

The district nurse meets many elderly people who have dental problems, of which one is that their gums have receded so that the dentures no longer stay in place. They continue to wear them, developing mouth ulcers which in turn lead to a poor appetite.

Some elderly people manage to chew meat and fruit quite adequately with their gums and do not appear to need or want dentures. Others resort to soft foods which may not provide the required nutrients. Some patients will have some of their own teeth which are loose and carious and their gums may be unhealthy – all reasons for the district nurse to try and persuade her patient to visit a dentist. She must remember that sore lips and buccal mucosa may be due to a candida infection, but a sore tongue should alert her to the possibility of pernicious anaemia.

CARE OF THE FEET

Painful corns and long toenails (which may become ingrown due to lack of attention) are a common cause of decreased mobility. This may be due to the fact that the patient is too obese or crippled with arthritis to cut his toenails, or possibly to self-neglect. A patient suffering from onychogryphosis will have nails that are long, twisted and horn-like, and may not have been touched for two or more years. This condition cannot wait for a chiropodist to be contacted, and the nurse must deal with it immediately. The feet should be given a lengthy soaking in a bowl of warm water and then nail clippers used on the softened toenails.

When bathing or washing a patient, the nurse should ensure that the feet are dried well, especially between the toes, and then powdered carefully. Toenails should be kept short and cut straight across; the patient should be encouraged to wear shoes which fit well for walking. The services of a qualified chiropodist are needed if a patient is suffering from corns, callosities, bunions or other foot deformities.

SLEEP AND INSOMNIA

Many elderly people sleep for only short periods. Some go to bed early after a relatively inactive day and worry because they cannot get to sleep. The nurse should reassure them that sleeplessness is not harmful, since they do not need as much sleep as a person leading an active life. She may suggest they take a warm, milky drink before bed, possibly with some alcohol in it; stress that they go to the lavatory before retiring, and to make themselves as warm and comfortable as possible in bed. Sometimes reading a light novel may induce sleep or listening to a quiet radio programme. Symptoms such as pain and dyspnoea are not conducive to sleep, and specific medical treatment and possibly the use of a backrest and bedcradle are needed in some cases. The GP may eventually prescribe sleeping tablets and ask the district nurse to monitor the effectiveness of the chosen drug. The patient is advised not to take his sleeping tablet until he has got into bed, otherwise he is liable to go to sleep in a chair, and then, later in the night, sustains a fall when, half-awake, he attempts to go to bed. He is also told not to keep his bottle of sleeping tablets on the bedside table in case, later in the night, he should inadvertently take a second or third tablet.

FALLS

Falls are more dangerous for an elderly person than for a younger individual as old bones are brittle and fracture more easily yet take longer to heal. Some of the causes of falls in the elderly are shown in Figure 8/2. Falls due to faults in the environment call for the practice of preventive medicine by the district nurse.

Accidental falls may be avoided by:

(a) Removing loose mats from slippery floors.
(b) Putting up extra banisters (or handrails).
(c) Improving the lighting of dimly lit halls and passageways.
(d) Removing the hazard of trailing flexes and fixing carpet rods on the staircase.
(e) Obtaining a commode to place beside the bed and so remove the need to leave the bedroom at night.
(f) Converting a downstairs room into a bed-sitting room for a disabled patient thus avoiding the dangers of stairs.
(g) Encouraging old people to walk with support from a solid object.

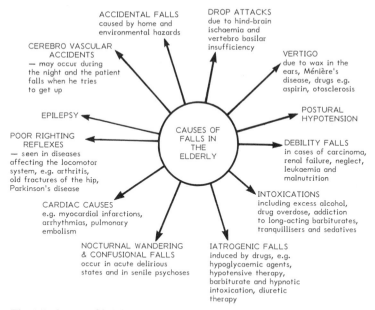

Fig. 8/2 Causes of falls in the elderly

(h) Enlisting the help of the social services department with home conversion and adaptation to make a safer environment. Local voluntary groups are often willing to decorate and adapt the houses of the elderly.

(i) Arranging a visit to the optician if the patient's eyesight appears defective, as the provision of spectacles may help to prevent falls.

(j) Arranging regular chiropody treatment for patients immobilised by painful corns and bunions.

Voluntary organisations such as Age Concern play an important part in encouraging and promoting safety for the elderly, and the district nurse may refer to them for advice if local authority help is not forthcoming.

HYPOTHERMIA

The dangers of hypothermia in the elderly have been much

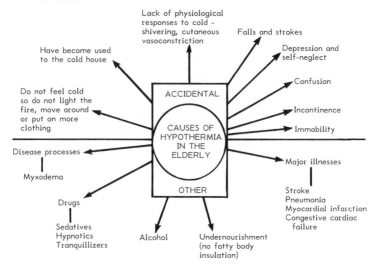

Fig. 8/3 Causes of hypothermia in the elderly

publicised in recent years and the Health Education Council runs a campaign annually, stressing the dangers of the condition and how to prevent its occurrence. In hypothermia, the core temperature of the body falls below 35°C (95°F) and the two most common causes are low environmental temperature and a defective temperature regulating system in the brain. Figure 8/3 shows accidental and other causes of hypothermia.

Prevention

The district nurse must pay particular attention to patients who fall into an at-risk category. A rectal temperature check using a low-reading thermometer is the best way of confirming whether a patient is reaching a state of hypothermia; it is an insurance against a missed diagnosis which could be fatal.

Adequate and sensible clothing is essential for the elderly especially during the winter months. If they cannot afford warm clothes the district nurse may obtain blankets and clothing from the local WRVS clothing store. The social worker must be told that there is a person at risk of hypothermia so that she can visit and arrange for extra heating, meals on wheels, and perhaps a home help or good neighbour to call and keep an eye on the patient, giving plenty of hot drinks. The nurse must try and persuade the patient to have heating in his bedroom and not leave the window open at night. Mobility should be encouraged.

Clinical features

The elderly person does not look cold however cold the room seems to the visitor. His hands and face look red and warm but feel cold. The speech may be slow and slurred, the pulse slow, and he may be confused or drowsy, but does not shiver. His abdomen and the insides of the thighs are icy cold and clammy. The rectal temperature is subnormal, respirations slow and shallow, the blood pressure drops and the muscles go into spasm as his condition deteriorates.

Management

In most cases hospital admission is essential. The aim is to re-warm the patient at the rate of 0.5 to 1°C hourly by wrapping him in blankets and nursing him in a room temperature of 25°C. Hot-water bottles must *not* be used as they cause vasodilatation and a further drop in blood pressure. If conscious, frequent warm drinks are given.

Once a patient has been treated for hypothermia in hospital, he should not be discharged into the same cold environment until conditions have been rectified.

DEFICIENCY DISEASES

Iron deficiency anaemia

The onset of iron deficiency anaemia is often an insidious process and one taken for granted by many old people, who accept tiredness, weakness and breathlessness as part of getting old. The two main causes are faulty dietary habits and bleeding. The GP will arrange various investigations once anaemia is diagnosed and the district nurse may help by taking blood for a full blood count and collecting specimens of faeces for occult blood. Iron tablets may be prescribed or the district nurse may be asked to visit to give iron by injection in a dose calculated to replace the deficiency and leave reserves for the future. This is given intramuscularly (in the form of an iron-dextran complex) and the nurse uses a Z-shaped injection technique to prevent leakage of the solution back into the subcutaneous tissue and thus staining of the skin. The injection must be given deep into the muscle to prevent superficial abscess formation.

Z-shaped technique: This necessitates moving the subcutaneous layer of skin to one side before injecting, and allowing it to spring back afterwards, giving a Z-shaped injection channel.

If the cause of the anaemia is shown to be dietary, the nurse will need to spend time with her patient discussing what should be included in the daily diet.

Pernicious anaemia

Pernicious anaemia is due to a lack of vitamin B_{12} which is needed to produce normal red blood cells. Over half the patients who develop this condition are elderly. Typical symptoms include those of anaemia, a tingling sensation in the hands and feet (due to subacute combined degeneration of the spinal cord), a smooth glossy tongue and a yellowish tint to the skin. Once diagnosed, these patients will become part of the district nurse's regular caseload as they need maintenance injections for the rest of their lives. The usual time interval between injections is eight weeks for Neo-Cytamen as it is excreted more slowly, and two to four weeks for Cytamen which is excreted more rapidly. A test dose should be administered initially by the district nurse who is trained to deal with anaphylactic shock (see p. 161) should it occur.

Osteoporosis

In osteoporosis, the bone structure is normal, but the amount of bone present is reduced and fractures are a risk. The patient complains of bone pain, particularly in the back; the vertebrae may collapse leading to kyphosis.

The district nurse can help by encouraging mobility, because old bones lose calcium when a patient is immobile and will not strengthen nor regain their calcium unless put to proper weight-bearing use. She will also stress the importance of a nutritious diet containing plenty of milk and bread. The doctor may prescribe calcium tablets, and analgesics if the patient is in pain. A corset may help severe back pain. The nurse must also advise the patient and his family on how to remove or remedy home hazards which could cause the patient to fall.

Osteomalacia

This condition is often confused with osteoporosis. It is known that the softening of the bones which occurs in osteomalacia is due to a lack of vitamin D or its metabolites impairing the calcification of the bones. Treatment is replacement therapy. The patient might have become immobile due to pain in his hips, thighs, shoulders or back. He may have had difficulty in climbing stairs, and his hip movements are weak as well as painful leading to a 'waddling gait'.

Treatment usually commences with a parenteral injection of 600 000 units of calciferol although some doctors prefer oral therapy. The district nurse may be asked to carry out regular venepuncture for serum calcium estimations to ensure that hypercalcaemia does not occur. She should also advise on diet and the need for more fresh air and exposure to sunlight.

Hypothyroidism

Hypothyroidism (myxoedema) is a fairly common condition among the elderly, and because of its gradual onset it is often overlooked and mistaken for the effects of ageing. It is more common in elderly women and is rare in a male. The patient slows down in speech, movements and reactions. She is mildly confused and often constipated. Her skin appears cold, dry and pale; her hair is thin and brittle, and her face puffy especially around the eyes. Her voice deepens and becomes hoarser. As the bodily processes have slowed down there is the added danger of hypothermia.

Diagnosis is confirmed by blood tests to estimate the amount of circulating thyroid hormone, and treatment is by oral thyroxine, starting with a very small daily dose, gradually increasing to a maintenance dose. If the heart is sound when the GP examines her she is started on thyroxine at home under the supervision of the district nurse.

DISABLING DISEASES

Both osteoarthritis and rheumatoid arthritis are frequently seen when the district nurse visits elderly people and these are discussed in Chapter 9.

Parkinson's disease

Parkinson's disease is a chronic and distressing condition, both for the patient and his family as it affects speech and co-ordination. It is a disease of later life, starting insidiously about 60 to 70 years and ending in disability. Clinical features include hypokinesia, tremor, muscular rigidity and mental disturbances.

It is often difficult to nurse a case of Parkinson's disease at home and a careful assessment and much support is needed. The district nurse usually meets her patient and his relatives in the early stages of the disease when all that is needed is advice, mobilisation of resources and possibly help with bathing. At this time the patient should be encouraged to take regular exercise, but not to the point of fatigue. Warm baths are helpful. Inactivity for too long makes for immobility. Physiotherapy is important and the physiotherapist will advise about exercise programmes. Relatives should be encouraged to co-operate so that exercises can be continued at home with 'refresher' visits to the physiotherapy department. The district nurse can help in encouraging the patient (and family) to follow the programme. If necessary a joint visit by the district nurse and the occupational therapist can help to identify problems of self-care within the patient's home. Various aids and handrails can then be provided.

Drug therapy

There are drugs available which have changed the outlook for some patients suffering from Parkinson's disease. With parkinsonism there is too little dopamine and too much acetylcholine in the brain, which affects the transmission of nerve impulses. Treatment is therefore aimed at replacing the dopamine and reducing the acetylcholine.

Levodopa (L-Dopa): Levodopa is effective in all forms of the disease and may be used at any stage to lessen rigidity, akinesia and tremor. In most patients the benefits last for two or three years. Adverse effects to be observed by the district nurse include transient mental confusion, abnormality of heart rhythm and sometimes abnormal facial movements.

Amantadine (Symmetrel): If the patient cannot tolerate levodopa, amantadine is often prescribed.

Anti-cholinergic drugs: These were used in the treatment of parkinsonism prior to the introduction of levodopa. They are still used as an alternative if levodopa is not tolerated and sometimes used with it. Side-effects include blurred vision, constipation, retention of urine and delirium.

Nursing care

Initially, all that is needed from the district nurse is support and advice, coupled with observation of the patient's progress and ensuring that the carers are managing to cope. She may arrange for one of her team to help the patient bath each week. The district nurse will advise the family about his diet which should include plenty of fluids and be high in calories (tremor and rigidity result in raised metabolic demands). Constipation is often a problem so extra roughage is needed in the patient's diet and laxatives may need to be prescribed by the GP.

In the final stages of the disease much nursing care and help is needed. Pressure-area care is vital. Incontinence may occur placing an extra strain on family resources. The patient needs to be fed, which is a slow and laborious process. He will only be able to take soft foods because he finds swallowing difficult due to excessive salivation and muscular weakness. There is often difficulty in changing the patient's pyjamas because of contracted limbs, and in cleaning his teeth if they are tightly clenched. Some dementia may be present. While the district nurse may visit two or three times a day, she must be aware of the strain placed on the family who are 'on duty' 24 hours a day, seven days a week. She must therefore seek help from social services for the family and if a night-sitter service exists it too should be requested. In some areas a shared-care service exists whereby the patient can spend two weeks in hospital and six or more weeks at home. This gives the family a welcome break from caring. In some cases where the family is unable to provide the necessary care and support then admission to a long-stay ward is the only solution.

PSYCHOLOGICAL PROBLEMS IN THE ELDERLY

Loneliness

Loneliness is a very real problem among the elderly. It may be the underlying cause of many conditions the district nurse encounters, especially self-neglect and malnutrition. Factors responsible for this problem are shown in Figure 8/4.

Many lonely old people rely on the visits of the district nurse to break the monotony of their day. An old lady may deliberately scratch her legs to cause a breakdown in the healing of her ulcers

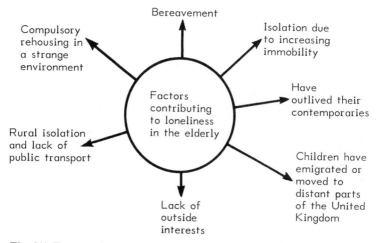

Fig. 8/4 Factors which may lead to loneliness in the elderly

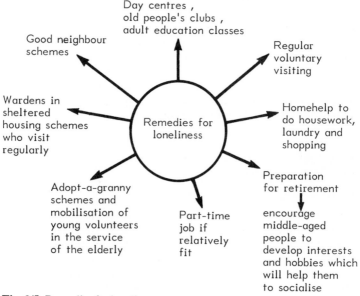

Fig. 8/5 Remedies for loneliness

when the district nurse starts to reduce her visits. Figure 8/5 shows some remedies to the problems of loneliness in the elderly.

Mental confusion

In an elderly patient confusion of sudden onset is more often than not a sign of physical illness, and if the cause is treated the condition is reversible. The patient is usually confused concerning facts and the identity of people, is likely to be disorientated in time and space, and hallucinations may occur, as may a noisy delirium which often fluctuates with lucid intervals.

Conditions which predispose to mental confusion in the elderly include:

(a) Infections of the respiratory or urinary tract where fever is often absent, and in the elderly confusion may be the first symptom observed.
(b) Minor strokes causing temporary confusion.
(c) Any disease which deprives the brain of oxygen, for example, anaemia, cardiac failure, acute bronchitis, hypotension, shock and hypothermia.
(d) Postoperatively following general anaesthesia.
(e) The effect of drugs such as digoxin, barbiturates, hypotensive drugs and alcohol.
(f) Uraemia, dehydration, sepsis and thyrotoxicosis.

Management of mental confusion

Once the cause of the confusion has been found, the relatives can be reassured that it is only a temporary condition which will resolve with treatment, and advised to approach the patient with calmness and reassurance. The aim is to keep down the emotional temperature and to prevent arguments. The patient needs company and people with time to talk to him, rather than being given sedatives which would probably aggravate the confusional state. If the relatives can cope, then the patient is best cared for at home, as admission to hospital tends to exaggerate confusion. He should not be forcibly restrained. He needs to be helped to the lavatory at regular intervals and any constipation problems should be reported to the nurse.

Dementia

Dementia is probably due to arteriosclerosis or to actual physical changes in the brain leading to atrophy of brain cells. The most usual group (aged 75 to 85) first become forgetful, have accidents, forget their shopping and generally neglect themselves. They may have memory lapses for recent events, yet remember things which happened in their childhood. They lose articles, forgetting where they have put them. Gradual deterioration occurs and they are unable to dress themselves. They become incontinent, first of urine, then of faeces, and eventually cannot feed themselves or find their way around the house.

Management of dementia

The care of a patient with dementia (whose relatives wish to care for him at home) is largely supportive. A discussion with the relatives is essential, so that they know what to expect should the patient's condition deteriorate. At first living at home is beneficial, the surroundings are familiar and the routine known. It is important for the patient to be occupied so that he does not become isolated in his room away from family and reality. He should be encouraged to read newspapers and books, and to wear spectacles if he is accustomed to do so. Boredom must be avoided. Elderly confused patients are particularly sensitive to disapproval and respond to affection.

Where home safety is concerned, the patient should, if possible, sleep in a room downstairs. All fires should be guarded and medicines stored in a locked cupboard and given to the patient by a member of the family at the appropriate time. He needs regular nourishing meals, with plenty of fruit, vegetables and meat for their iron, vitamin and roughage content. Nocturnal restlessness may be due to discomfort caused by a full bladder or rectum and relatives should be aware of this possibility. If insomnia is a problem, then the patient should be given a warm milky drink with a little alcohol added if he desires. If these remedies fail, the GP must be consulted, and he may prescribe a hypnotic, for example dichloralphenazone (Welldorm) which is particularly suitable for confused elderly patients.

Relatives need much respite when caring for the demented, and day care facilities should be requested for two or three days a week in order to give them a rest, and the patient may be admitted into residential care several times a year so that the family can take a holiday.

When the strain of caring becomes too great, long-term admission to a special home for the 'elderly mentally infirm' or psychiatric hospital care should be considered.

Depression

The elderly often have many reasons for depression including:

Problems of deafness or blindness
Pain due to arthritis
Recent bereavement
Financial problems
Children grown up and living at a distance, unable to visit frequently
Failure of health and mobility
A feeling of being unwanted and a burden on family and society.

If the depression occurs as a result of their reaction to a distressing episode, then the support of friends and relatives, and help from supportive statutory services may help them pull through without medical help.

The district nurse is often one of the most frequent visitors to the homes of the elderly. She plays many roles apart from that of a professional highly qualified nurse. She is a friend and confidante; a supporter and adviser to patient and family; a liaison link with (and co-ordinator of) other services; a teacher and health educator and a member of the team of people providing care for the elderly.

BIBLIOGRAPHY

Anderson, F. W., Caird, F. I., Kennedy, R. D. and Schwartz, D. (1983). *Gerontology and Geriatric Nursing*. Hodder and Stoughton, Sevenoaks.

Awdry, P. and Nicholls, C. S. (1985). *Cataract*. Faber and Faber, London.

Carver, V. and Liddiard, P. (jt eds) (1978). *An Ageing Population*. Hodder and Stoughton, Sevenoaks in association with the Open University Press.

Hawker, M. (1985). *The Older Patient and the Role of the Physiotherapist*. Faber and Faber, London.

Leydhecker, W. and Pitts Crick, R. (1981). *All About Glaucoma: Questions and Answers for People with Glaucoma.* Faber and Faber, London.

Wilcock, G. K. and Middleton, A. M. (1980). *Geriatrics.* Grant McIntyre Medical and Scientific, London.

Chapter Nine

THE PHYSICALLY HANDICAPPED PATIENT

In this chapter the term physically handicapped is used to encompass not only the arthritic patient but also those who have undergone amputation of a limb; or are paralysed either as the result of traumatic paraplegia or through a chronic illness such as multiple sclerosis. The physically disabled and their families often need help, advice and nursing care from the district nurse. The Government Report (1976) *'Priorities for Health and Personal Social Services in England'* stated that services for the physically handicapped needed to expand by 9 per cent per year. The district nurse should be aware of the help available in her area for industrial rehabilitation or vocational training and whether a disablement resettlement officer (DRO) is based at the local Job Centre. She will also need to know what statutory community services for the disabled are available and which voluntary organisations provide help and advice.

MAIN LEGISLATION CONCERNED WITH THE DISABLED

The National Assistance Act 1948

This Act empowered local authorities to help 'persons who are blind, deaf or dumb, and others substantially and permanently handicapped by illness, injury, congenital deformity, or other such disability as may be prescribed by the Minister'. This help may include:

Advice on services available
Provision of recreational facilities
Compilation and maintenance of a register
Provision of work

Provision of workshops and help in marketing the products therefrom

Provision of hostels

Instruction in ways of overcoming the effects of a disability.

The Chronically Sick and Disabled Persons Act 1970

This Act has greatly extended provisions for the handicapped. The Act lays down specific services which social services departments must provide for severely disabled people, including provision of telephones, aids and adaptations, holidays, etc. At the same time it gives the local authority the discretion to decide who is eligible for these services.

The Social Services Act 1970

This Act aimed to unify personal social services including:

(a) Home services: home helps, meals on wheels, transport to and from clubs and day centres run by the social services; car badges for the disabled to allow parking; provision of telephone, wireless, and television in some cases; help with special holiday needs
(b) Home adaptations: ramps, grab rails and other alterations
(c) Aids and equipment for daily living, bathing, toilet aids, hoists and walking frames
(d) Short- and long-term residential care
(e) Day centres and clubs to provide light work, diversionary activities and companionship
(f) Support from a social work team.

REHABILITATION

The aim of all rehabilitation is independence for the individual patient, according to his capabilities. The district nurse will help to achieve this and in so doing will find herself working as a member of a team which includes doctors, physiotherapists, occupational therapists, speech therapists, remedial gymnasts, social workers, technicians, voluntary workers, together with the patient and his family. As well as helping the patient achieve physical independence the team will need to sustain the family and see that they allow the patient to be fully involved in all decisions affecting his recovery.

It is often the district nurse who is consulted about financial entitlements and she should be able to advise on how and where to get further information about this (see pp. 188–9).

Aids for daily living

These are the responsibility of the local authority and the need for them will be assessed by the occupational therapist. If practical, it may be possible to arrange a visit to the nearest demonstration centre where a large range of aids can be tried (see DLF, p. 193). These include a split level cooker, lever type handles for water taps or possibly a simple tap turner. Electric power points should be installed commensurate with the height of the patient and easy-to-grip plugs are usually available. Cutlery with wider handles is available to a patient whose grip is weak. An electric kettle (with automatic cut-out device) can be fitted to a tilter base to save lifting. The patient should choose lightweight saucepans with a handle on both sides and, by using a saucepan strainer inside the pan, the lifting of heavy pans can be avoided.

Lavatories may be fitted with raised seats and grab rails according to the patient's need. Bath boards, seats and non-slip mats, together with fitted grab rails, help disabled patients to bath. Hoists can be fitted in a bedroom or bathroom for a paraplegic patient. Showers are preferable for the disabled, and are often incorporated in specially designed housing. Long-handled brushes or sponges may help the handicapped to wash themselves.

Transport

This is an individual matter but of vital importance to a handicapped person. Suitable modifications of the patient's own car may be made. The orange badge scheme for disabled drivers or passengers gives exemption from time-limits on parking meters and may allow parking on a single yellow line, providing obstruction is not caused.

Various wheelchairs with attachments and fittings are available to suit a patient's needs and disability. Some fold to fit in a car boot, others are powered by 6- to 12-volt batteries for persons unable to propel an ordinary wheelchair. Applications for *permanent* wheelchairs should be made by the patient's general practitioner to the nearest artificial limb and appliance centre. The British Red Cross Society provide wheelchairs on a loan basis for a period of six months.

Group transport is provided by the social services department to carry the handicapped to various centres. Some of these vehicles have side or rear hydraulic lifts which allow the patient to remain seated in his wheelchair. Voluntary organisations may run clubs and day centres while being supported and financed by the local authority who provides transport. Other facilities include hairdressing, occupational therapy and chiropody.

THE DISTRICT NURSE AND THE DISABLED

Patients with rheumatoid arthritis

Rheumatoid arthritis is a chronic inflammatory disease of unknown cause, which affects certain joints and organs of the body. Its course is one of exacerbation and remission, the amount of eventual handicap being influenced by the quality of care given during the acute exacerbations of the disease. At such a time the patient is usually admitted to hospital where attention to details such as position of the joints and appropriate splintage is of long-term importance.

The district nurse will visit those patients who need nursing care because of the disease or because they are bedridden. Medical care of the patient is directed towards the suppression of the inflammatory process by drugs; the physiotherapist will advise how best to prevent deformities by correct positioning and splinting as well as by the maintenance and promotion of joint function.

Drugs

The district nurse will observe and recognise any side-effects of the anti-inflammatory drugs prescribed and check the dosage. Salicylates, such as aspirin, may cause gastro-intestinal upsets, heartburn and, in high doses, tinnitus and deafness. In patients with peptic ulcers, haemorrhage from the gastric mucosa could occur.

Synthetic corticosteroids may be prescribed if the disease is progressing, is painful, and has not responded to other drugs. Oral steroids are available in an enteric-coated form to lessen the risk of gastro-intestinal irritation. If oral steroids are not tolerated the district nurse may be asked by the general practitioner to give injections of adrenocorticotrophic hormone (ACTH) at regular weekly, fortnightly or monthly intervals. When administering this drug, the nurse must be aware of the danger of hypersensitivity to the animal protein in the preparation and the possibility of anaphylactic shock.

Gold is an effective long-term anti-inflammatory agent used in the treatment of rheumatoid arthritis. It is given by injection as sodium aurothiomalate (Myocrisin), and the dosage will be prescribed by the rheumatologist. Side-effects of gold injections can be severe and occur in about one-third of patients. Before giving the injection the nurse must inspect the patient's skin for rashes and test his urine for protein, because skin, kidneys and bone marrow can be affected. Weekly blood counts should also be taken. Gold injections must be stopped and the doctor informed if any of the above-mentioned side-effects occur. Health authorities require their district nursing sisters to undergo a course of instruction in the procedure of venepuncture before attempting it in the patient's home (see p. 185).

Patients with rheumatoid arthritis may become anaemic due to iron deficiency. The district nurse may be asked to give iron injections using the Z-track injection technique (see p. 96) to prevent staining of the skin.

The nurse's first visit

The initial referral may be for a regular weekly injection as mentioned above. Whatever the reason, on the first visit the district nurse should assess the home situation. Her aim will be to discover if anything further can be done to improve the comfort of the patient, or to ease his mode of living. She will liaise with any agencies who may be involved. A plan of nursing care will be discussed with the patient and his family, or if he lives alone then she may need to call on the community support services. Patients with rheumatoid arthritis are often underweight so the nurse will need to advise on a high calorie diet with vitamin supplements to stimulate the appetite. If the patient needs help with personal hygiene, this too is planned and an offer made for a member of the nursing team to bath the patient once weekly. The nurse should stress to the patient and his family the need to keep a balance between rest and exercise.

If the patient is confined to bed a daily visit may be needed to help him wash and to attend to his pressure areas. If painful joints are immobilised by the application of splints, these should be removed daily so that the limbs can be washed and powdered.

Depending on local practice, and if the nurse has been taught how, active, assisted exercises can be carried out. As the acute inflammation subsides, independence and active exercises are encouraged. Exercises are of value only if carried out regularly and the nurse should encourage the patient. Heat, in the form of a pad or a covered hot-water bottle applied to the painful joints, helps to reduce pain and muscle spasm. On the other hand it may be inappropriate for some patients. Care must be taken not to burn the patient.

Nursing care of a patient with rheumatoid arthritis presents certain problems. The patient may have been ill for a long time; he may be worried, irritable, impatient or discouraged. Progress may be slow. The district nurse must help the patient to set himself realistic goals and encourage him that progress is being made. When nursing him during acute exacerbations of the disease she must be patient and unhurried, avoiding jarring and quick, jerky movements. Psychological support is very important and the nurse must be ready to listen to her patient's problems. Sources of concern to the patient include restricted employment, reduced earning capacity and limited social and recreational activities. The nurse may ask the social worker for help and advice in these matters, if the patient is willing.

The patient may have had recent surgery to relieve the symptoms of arthritis, and the district nurse may then be asked to dress the wound and remove the sutures. The common surgical procedures would be arthrodesis (stiffening of the joint), arthroplasty (joint replacement) and the removal of rheumatic nodules.

Patients with osteoarthritis

Rheumatoid arthritis can develop at any time from childhood to old age; osteoarthrosis is primarily a disease of older age-groups. It is a disease of the joints alone as opposed to a systemic disease, and sometimes only one joint is involved. The patient complains of stiffness, soreness and pain in the affected joints and his range of movement becomes increasingly limited. Crepitus may be heard or felt on movement.

Care of the patient

The patient is usually treated with medication and physiotherapy. If obese, he will be encouraged to lose weight to reduce the strain on his painful joints. Simple analgesics such as aspirin and benorylate are commonly prescribed. Appropriate exercises may be taught to strengthen and maintain muscle tone and to increase the range of movement.

Work should be interspersed with periods of rest, and unnecessary walking, lifting, stair climbing and bending avoided. Good posture should be encouraged. If the disease involves the hip joint the patient should be advised to lie on his bed in the prone position for an hour morning and evening to prevent worsening of the flexion deformity of the hip. Disease in this joint is particularly disabling and the patient may have problems in using the lavatory and in sexual activities. Getting up from a low chair can be a slow, laborious process, but the social services department can provide a high seated chair, a raised lavatory seat and grab rails for the lavatory and bathroom. Other aids include a pick-up stick (Helping Hand), a stocking aid and a walking stick or Zimmer frame. Chiropody is often essential. As with rheumatoid arthritis, the application of heat pads may help relieve the pain.

A person below retirement age may need to change jobs because of the disabling effects of the disease. The disablement resettlement officer may be able to help. Strenuous sports and other forms of recreation may also have to be given up, and less energetic hobbies cultivated. Arthroplasty (or arthrodesis) may be advised by the orthopaedic surgeon.

Total hip replacement

This is the usual type of arthroplasty carried out. Postoperatively the time of mobilisation depends upon the preference of the surgeon. The patient is often discharged home within two weeks and in some cases the district nurse may be asked to remove the sutures. Psychological support is essential when the patient comes home as he suffered much pain and disability before the operation and now needs repeated assurance that he can rely on the new joint to walk comfortably and securely. A few patients who have had a hip arthroplasty may need to continue to attend physiotherapy sessions to help their final rehabilitation. The district nurse should check that the patient can walk up and down stairs, dress himself and get in and out of the bath with minimal assistance. If he has problems the nurse should talk to the appropriate team member regarding help.

The amputee

Each year about 5000 new patients are referred to artificial limb and appliance centres (ALACs), and 4500 of these are lower limb amputees. Many are elderly.

Before discharge of an amputee it is almost essential that the district nurse and the domiciliary occupational therapist are told, so that any equipment required is provided, and if necessary, help from the community support services organised. The living accommodation may have to be adapted to suit his immediate needs after which a long-term plan can be made. If the house is too small or the stairs unnegotiable, he may need to apply for rehousing. Home hazards such as trailing flexes, slip mats and obstructive furniture must be removed to prevent the patient from injuring himself.

If both the patient and his family are elderly it might mean that initially a member of the district nursing team will have to visit daily to help the patient out of bed and attend to his hygiene needs. Care of his pressure areas must also be carried out and exercises encouraged.

Care of the stump

Opinions vary as to the benefits of stump bandaging. The nurse will be advised as to the practice of individual units or surgeons.

Once the patient has a prosthesis he should wear a stump sock, which must fit well, be wrinkle free and changed daily. If the stump becomes red, swollen or irritates, the patient must stop wearing his prosthesis and report the problem to his doctor. Limb fitting centres will advise on specific problems and the district nurse should make herself conversant with the preferred approach to care and rehabilitation.

The recent amputee should not sit for too long in low soft chairs. A suitable regime, before obtaining the prosthesis, would be – two hours in a comfortable chair, two hours on a hard-backed chair with the chair facing the bed, and then an hour lying supine on the bed to prevent flexion deformities. A position facing the bed provides a suitable surface for reading matter and a food tray. The patient should also be encouraged to lean on the bed and raise himself up on to the sound leg. This relieves pressure and strengthens the leg muscles.

Throughout the rehabilitation period, emphasis on perseverance should be important. Considerable physical effort is needed and this may lead to despondency. The nurse and rehabilitation team must set attainable goals, encouraging and praising the patient as he achieves each step. It is hoped that, with the help of the disablement resettlement officer, the younger patient will return to work.

COMMUNITY CARE OF THE PARALYSED

Following spinal injury, it is usual for the patient to be admitted to a specialist centre such as Stoke Mandeville. The initial admission period will be at least six months, and during this time the medical social worker will be liaising with the family and local authority to ensure that the patient's home conditions are adapted to suit his needs. The family may have to be rehoused. She also contacts the disablement resettlement officer to plan the patient's possible return to employment after rehabilitation. The ward sister usually informs the district nurse of the patient's impending discharge and suggests that she may wish to visit him in hospital to note the relevant nursing techniques used in his particular case. Optimum independence is the aim.

When the district nurse carries out her first home assessment following discharge she must remember that it is the prevention (or early treatment) of potential problems such as pressure sores, chest infections, contractures, urinary tract infections, or other bladder and bowel problems, which is so important.

Pressure sores

Paraplegics and tetraplegics are more vulnerable to pressure because of loss of sensation and lowered tissue resistance resulting from the vasomotor paralysis. The necessary preventive knowledge must be imparted to the patient and his family. The patient, and his family (if relevant), will have been thoroughly taught about looking after pressure areas, and the district nurse should only have to *remind* him of the importance of regular turns and lifts. For instance, the paraplegic with a four-inch thick sorbo rubber cushion in his chair is taught to lift his buttocks clear of the cushion for 20 seconds. This should be done every 10 to 15 minutes, and with practice should become an automatic procedure. Later he should be able to inspect his own pressure areas night and morning using a mirror. The tetraplegic can be provided with a ripple cushion for his chair. However, regular lifting to relieve pressure on *his* buttocks is still of vital importance and will need to be done by the *carer*. His pressure areas must be checked daily to ensure that no red areas are developing. The nurse must stress the importance of relieving all pressure on areas which develop blemishes until healing has occurred. This may mean a period of bedrest on a full-length sheepskin or an alternating pressure mattress, as these sores take a long time to heal if neglected.

Skin care is an essential part of the preventive process. The skin should be kept clean and dry. Talcum powder should be used sparingly as it can form granules, and if the patient's skin is moist, cause irritation. If the skin is dry, oil or lanolin may be useful especially on the soles of the feet where dead epithelium collects (if left it causes cracks to form). This may be seen on the palms of the tetraplegic.

Most paralysed patients and their carers have been thoroughly instructed prior to discharge in the procedures and routines necessary to prevent complications from occurring and to enable the patient to lead as independent a life as possible. The district nurse must reinforce those instructions. Particular emphasis must be placed on:

1. Passive exercises to the affected joints twice daily to prevent stiffening of the muscles and joints. This also helps to improve the circulation.
2. Scrupulous attention to bladder management to prevent infection and maintain a satisfactory emptying of the bladder so that residual urine is less than 100ml and any incontinence controlled. Any signs of infection must be reported immediately. The district nurse should remind the patient to drink at least 3 litres of fluid per day and check that he is coping with any appliances supplied by the hospital.
3. Bowel management which has been worked out in hospital. The district nurse must ensure that the carers and the patient are able to carry out the recommended routine.
4. The need for a high-protein, high-vitamin diet to promote tissue resistance and healing. Any tendency towards a negative nitrogen balance because of immobility, should be monitored.

The paraplegic patient should be able to carry out sedentary work; he has less problems than the tetraplegic who can only work under sheltered conditions, if at all. Most tetraplegics are provided with an electric wheelchair which can be adapted to the individual person's needs. An aid such as POSSUM can contribute considerably to the independence of a severely disabled patient.

Paralysis is a terrible shock to a person. The individual reaction to the loss of function varies. Many patients go through a stage of denial, others become very depressed. The patient must be encouraged to partake fully in his rehabilitation, for it is his own effort that is needed to achieve independence. The district nurse plays her part in what is a team effort by helping him to manage both his physical problems and normal activities of living when discharged from the security of the hospital environment.

CARE OF THE PATIENT WITH MULTIPLE SCLEROSIS (MS)

Multiple sclerosis is a demyelinating disease with no specific cause. It may be relatively benign, or severe, leading to marked disability. It is the latter group of patients that the district nurse is more likely to meet.

The main aim when caring for a patient with MS is to keep him mobile for as long as possible. In the earlier stages of the disease, if vision is affected, the district nurse may be asked to visit to give injections of adrenocorticotrophic hormone (ACTH). Later she may become more involved as provision of general nursing care becomes more necessary.

As with the paralysed patient, confirmation of diagnosis comes as a shock and the reaction may be one of severe anxiety, anger or denial at first, and later depression. Given time the patient should adjust to his illness and accept its limitations. The nurse should encourage her patient to express this anger and frustration; and learn to overcome at least some of his problems and disabilities. She may put him in touch with the Multiple Sclerosis Society, which has visiting welfare officers.

Family problems

Multiple sclerosis can cause unhappiness within the family, especially between marriage partners and children. The nurse who visits the patient should understand, be sympathetic and be ready to talk about any problems. This is a valid reason for building up a good relationship with the patient and his family initially. A patient may fear that if too many demands are made on his partner he could face rejection; the partner may not wish to express anger for fear of hurting the ill person, and so on. Alternatively the patient may use illness to manipulate the family by inducing guilt, and they may over-protect him, while suppressing feelings of hostility and anger. They should all be encouraged to talk openly about their feelings and worries, and the nurse can extend a helping hand by explaining that the patient's mood swings are part of the illness. The atmosphere at home and at work should be as relaxed as possible.

General needs

The nurse should advise the patient on a routine balancing rest with activity. He must not allow himself to become over-tired. At least eight hours sleep at night is recommended. During an acute exacerbation of the disease, rest in bed is necessary or admission to hospital. Other useful advice includes the need to avoid obesity.

Occupational needs

Occupation plays a vital part in keeping up morale in any illness and especially so in a chronic, relapsing disease. It is important for the male to be able to maintain his position as breadwinner of the family for as long as possible and not lose his personal identity. However it is sensible to make an assessment of the work situation. Increasing fatigue is usually an earlier problem than disablement, and it is better to make plans for the future. A steady job which does not demand a great deal of energy is the most the patient should undertake. It is good to develop any creative talents and hobbies at an early stage, as the pleasure of achievement is an antidote to the depression which all too often occurs with degenerative diseases. The nurse can encourage the patient to live as normally as possible within his limitations.

A housewife with multiple sclerosis may need help in the home and various adaptations can be made enabling her to continue as a wife and mother. If she has a full-time job she may need to change to part-time employment, or give up work entirely, thus saving her limited energy for the family and home.

Bladder and bowel problems

Urgency of micturition may occur; this can be helped by atropine or Pro-Banthine which relax the detrusor muscle and increase the bladder capacity. Later, the patient may suffer a loss of sphincter control and incontinence will follow (see Chapter 10).

Constipation, as in other diseases, can be a problem and the patient should be advised to increase the fluid and roughage content of his diet.

Motor disability

In the early stages of the disease the patient may find that he becomes more clumsy and that his limbs feel heavy. He may become unsteady when walking, have a tremor or shake in either or both hands, and suffer from twitching or muscle spasm in an affected leg. Changes in sensation may occur in the body as well as the limbs. Home hazards such as slip mats, trailing flexes, footstools and other such articles should be removed. Floors should not be waxed. Handrails can be fitted, but when stairs become a problem the patient should live on the ground floor until the family can be rehoused in a bungalow or ground floor flat. If a wheelchair life has to be accepted by patient and family, the occupational therapist and physiotherapist can advise on additional features which can be attached to the chair, making life easier and maintaining independence.

If the patient has sufficient strength in his arms and trunk, he can be taught how to move himself from bed or lavatory to his wheelchair and back again. As his spasticity worsens, the family must be taught how to lift and move him without injuring themselves. A hoist can be obtained and the district nurse or occupational therapist will supervise its installation and teach the relatives how to use it correctly.

The patient and his family can also be shown how to reduce the development of contractures and deformities by suitable positioning.

Loss of sensation

In multiple sclerosis, damage to the sensory pathways can cause a loss of awareness to temperature, pain and pressure. The patient therefore must avoid prolonged pressure on susceptible areas and should be particularly careful not to injure his limbs. Hot-water bottles should be covered, and a bath thermometer used to check the temperature of the water before the patient gets in.

Skin and mouth care

As the bedbound patient becomes less able to care for himself his position should be changed two-hourly and his skin kept clean and dry. A sheepskin to lie on helps to prevent soreness. The weight of the bedclothes can be supported by a bedcradle. His teeth and mouth should be cleaned after meals as food may accumulate owing to difficulty in swallowing. He may also have difficulty in coughing up mucus, which predisposes to chest infections, and help with deep breathing and coughing will need to be taught.

The patient who has become crippled by multiple sclerosis may have to be admitted into hospital or residential care if the family cannot take the strain of caring for him at home.

All physically disabled patients need help from the caring team in order to achieve optimum independence. For some, such as the multiple sclerosis patients, this may first be short-term with more care and support ultimately being needed. Other handicapped people may become self-sufficient so that the care of the nursing team is no longer needed. Independence within the limit of their disability is the potential goal of all handicapped people.

REFERENCE

DHSS (1976). *Priorities for Health and Personal Social Services in England. A Consultative Document.* HMSO, London.

BIBLIOGRAPHY

Forsythe, E. (1979). *Living with Multiple Sclerosis.* Faber and Faber, London.

Graham, J. (1981). *Multiple Sclerosis – A Self-help Guide to its Management.* Thorsons, Wellingborough.

Kratz, C. (1978). *The Care of the Long-term Sick in the Community.* Churchill Livingstone, Edinburgh.

Handling the Handicapped: A Guide to the Lifting and Movement of Disabled People, 2nd edition. Woodhead-Faulkner Ltd, Cambridge in association with the Chartered Society of Physiotherapy.

Matthews, W. B. (1978). *Multiple Sclerosis – The Facts.* Oxford University Press, Oxford.

Tarling, C. (1980). *Hoists and Their Use.* William Heinemann Medical Books Ltd, London, for the Disabled Living Foundation.

Chapter Ten

BOWEL AND BLADDER PROBLEMS

With problems arising from conditions affecting the bladder or bowel, the sufferer may be too embarrassed to seek help. For example, the person with a stoma tries to conceal this fact from his workmates and other contacts; people suffering from incontinence attempt to conceal it; the younger woman will wear a sanitary towel continuously and wash out countless pairs of panties each day, while the older person tries to hide wet or soiled pads and clothing.

Little mention is made of incontinence in the professional training of doctors, nurses and social workers. Constipation is studied as a symptom of organic disease and yet it is frequently caused by incorrect diet and irregular bowel habits. Each year, in NHS hospitals in England and Wales, approximately 5000 people have a permanent colostomy constructed for rectal carcinoma, and approximately 300 people with chronic inflammatory disease of the bowel have an ileostomy formed. The hospital nurse will deal with the immediate pre- and postoperative care of stoma patients, and the district nurse will visit all such patients routinely, following discharge, to provide any continuing care.

CARE OF THE STOMA PATIENT IN THE COMMUNITY

The colostomy patient

The main reason for excision of the rectum and the creation of a colostomy, is carcinoma of the lower third of the rectum. Some patients are aware they have malignant disease, others believe that the operation was necessary to remove an 'ulcer'. The district nurse must be told by the ward sister on the patient's discharge, whether or not he knows the diagnosis. This will influence her approach to the patient. Many elderly people find it difficult to adapt to a colostomy, and may have a degree of intellectual impairment which prevents them from understanding the mechanism of a stoma. Some patients never come to terms with it. Others may view the stoma with great distaste, and fear that they are constantly dirty and emit an unpleasant smell. It is often the district nurse who must help the patient to come to terms with his disability, and deal with any problems that may arise. Relatives, who at first feel nothing but relief that he has survived a serious operation, are sometimes repulsed by their first sight of the stoma and what it entails. The district nurse will need to encourage their acceptance of the situation.

The ileostomy patient

Most patients who require an ileostomy will have been ill for a long time suffering from an inflammatory disease of the colon such as ulcerative colitis or Crohn's disease. They may face the prospect of a permanent ileostomy with many anxieties about work, hobbies, marriage and sex. A visit, pre- or postoperatively, by a member of the Ileostomy Association who has himself undergone the same operation can help to put the patient's fears and worries in perspective. Many areas now employ a stomatherapist who can provide valuable support for district nurses caring for stoma patients with particular problems.

The district nurse will visit the stoma patient as soon as he returns home and will continue to visit for as long as necessary.

The first visit

This is usually a lengthy visit so that the patient can gain confidence in the nurse's ability to deal with his problems and so establish a satisfactory rapport. It is essential that the nurse shows no repugnance at the sight of the stoma as this would destroy the patient's fragile self-confidence. She asks him about any previous illnesses, his occupation, leisure hours and hobbies. He is encouraged to resume his normal activities as soon as possible.

Housing

Stoma patients need an inside lavatory, a fixed bath and piped hot and cold water, but in some parts of the country the standards of housing are such that one or more of these basic amenities is lacking. The patient may request rehousing on medical grounds.

Bathing

The patient may have a bath or shower with the appliance in position. If faecal discharge is minimal, showering without the appliance is good for the skin, but all soap residue should be rinsed away, as this can interfere with the seal provided by the bag adhesive. The stoma should be dried by patting either with gauze or toilet tissues. Swimming should not be a problem. Some patients feel safer if they wear a piece of gauze under waterproof tape, or slip on a small adhesive security bag which is waterproof.

Diet

If the patient worries about his diet, every encouragement should be given to eat normally, discovering by trial and error the foods which should be avoided. New foods should be tried one at a time and in this way it is easy to find which causes problems. At first the ileostomist should eat little and often, then increase his intake as the stomach settles and the small intestine starts to take over the water-absorbing function. Foods such as beans, peas, broccoli, spinach, fruit, baked beans and onions, and those which are highly spiced have been known to cause loose motions and each should be tried separately to ascertain the effects. Spirits and wine usually cause no harm, but beer sometimes causes gas and diarrhoea. Some appliances incorporate a special filter which automatically releases flatus but traps the smell.

Diarrhoea, involving considerable water loss must be controlled. Ileostomists in particular can soon become dehydrated and lose too much sodium and potassium. If a bad attack of diarrhoea occurs the GP must be informed; the patient should return to a low-residue diet with added salt and increased fluid intake until the diarrhoea settles. Eggs, boiled rice and tapioca can help to encourage a formed stool. The doctor may prescribe a drug such as codeine phosphate.

Odour

This is a problem that stoma patients initially worry about. It is relatively simple to control if the patient uses one of the modern odour-resistant appliances, keeps it clean and changes it regularly. Deodorants such as Nilodor are obtainable to put in the stoma bag.

Appliances

There are two types of stoma bag, namely disposable and

permanent. The latter is secured to a flange cemented directly to the skin, and to change it a solvent has to be applied to loosen the cement. This type of bag can last up to six months and the patient should be supplied with two or three to use in rotation. This will provide ample time for washing, drying and airing each bag in turn. The bags can be left in position for three to seven days. However, more stoma patients are now using disposable no-cement bags, which can be changed daily if necessary. Ileostomy bags can be left for a longer period of time as they are emptied more easily. Disposable bags can be changed in a matter of a few minutes. They should be emptied, rinsed and wrapped in newspaper before disposal in the dustbin. Most local authorities provide a special collection for this type of item but, understandably, many patients refuse the service and prefer privacy.

In some patients the stoma may continue to shrink for several months after surgery, so a review of the fit of the appliance is necessary at regular intervals. Too large a gasket can lead to leakage and skin excoriation especially in an ileostomy. Too small a gasket can cause friction on the side of the stoma and produce ulcers. The ideal bag should allow about 31mm (⅛″) clearance round the stoma.

Care of the skin

Preventing skin problems is better than treating them. It cannot be over-emphasised that each time the stoma bag is changed the skin must be washed gently with mild soap and water and thoroughly dried. The patient should be told that the most frequent cause of skin irritation is the leakage of faecal discharge under the face-plate of an incorrectly attached appliance, so that this can be avoided.

If the skin becomes excoriated, the use of Stomahesive is invaluable as it promotes rapid healing and acts as a second skin upon which to place the appliance. If dermatitis is severe the doctor may prescribe a hydrocortisone cream which is usually effective.

Special cotton covers are marketed which slip over the disposable polythene stoma bags, and these help to prevent the bag from sticking to the abdominal skin in hot weather, thus causing intense irritation.

Patients who have a colostomy or ileostomy can apply for a certificate of exemption from prescription charges for equipment obtainable under the NHS. The patient should always keep a month's supply of appliances at home in case there is any unforseen delay in renewing the prescriptions. The hospital usually ensures that the stoma patient is given sufficient supplies to last him for a month and a list of equipment to order from his GP on prescription.

Sex, marriage and children

Many younger ileostomy patients may have established a good sexual relationship before the operation. Joint discussions to give advice, support and encouragement to both partners may well be all that is needed to help them adjust to the new situation; where impotence of the husband occurs following ano-rectal surgery marital breakdowns may result. SPOD (see p. 191) will offer help in counselling.

Many ileostomists have had successful pregnancies. Nevertheless, doctors recommend that the patient should wait a year before considering pregnancy.

Once the patient can manage his stoma and has accepted the necessary adjustments to his lifestyle, he is ready to be discharged from the care of the district nurse. However, he should not feel 'abandoned' and the nurse must ensure that the patient knows how to contact her should a crisis arise.

CARE OF THE CONSTIPATED PATIENT

Most people have their own patent remedy for constipation but do not consider how it works or how to prevent a recurrence. Constipation is often a problem with the elderly and can lead to complications such as incontinence, faecal impaction, confusion and occasionally large bowel obstruction.

The causes of constipation may either be organic and need medical treatment, or functional and responsive to the advice and care of the nurse (Fig. 10/1). Many elderly people believe that they must have a daily evacuation of their bowels and resort to the repeated use of laxatives. This leads to a loss of intestinal tone and a reduced peristaltic response to normal food residue, and so another dose of laxative is taken. In this way the colon is unable to regain its natural rhythmic response to normal faecal mass.

Once the underlying cause has been identified, the nurse must relieve the discomfort by administering an enema or suppositories

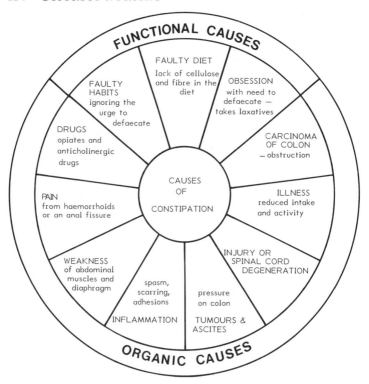

FUNCTIONAL CAUSES

FAULTY DIET
lack of cellulose
and fibre in the
diet

OBSESSION
with need to
defaecate —
takes laxatives

FAULTY
HABITS
ignoring the
urge to
defaecate

DRUGS
opiates and
anticholinergic
drugs

CARCINOMA
OF COLON
— obstruction

CAUSES
OF
CONSTIPATION

ILLNESS
reduced intake
and activity

PAIN
from haemorrhoids
or an anal fissure

INJURY OR
SPINAL CORD
DEGENERATION

WEAKNESS
of abdominal
muscles and
diaphragm

spasm,
scarring,
adhesions

pressure
on colon

INFLAMMATION

TUMOURS &
ASCITES

ORGANIC CAUSES

Fig. 10/1 Causes of constipation

and then try to educate the patient and his family as to how to prevent the condition from recurring.

Enemata and suppositories

It is more usual for district nurses to use disposable enemata such as phosphate or micralax enemata. On rare occasions she may be required to administer a one-pint soap and water enema and so most district nurses still have funnels, rubber tubing and disposable rectal catheters in their equipment bag. The procedure is the same as is carried out in hospital but there can be problems if the patient's toilet is outside or some distance from his bed. A commode or bedpan is useful.

Suppositories are not so drastic as enemata and can usually be retained for at least 20 minutes. Faecal impaction frequently occurs in older patients, and in those with disorders of the central nervous system. It may present as faecal incontinence with diarrhoea. In this case the nurse may first need to give an olive oil retention enema followed by a manual evacuation of faeces using a gloved finger. A small tap-water enema completes the procedure.

Once the constipation is treated, the nurse can discuss how to prevent its recurrence. Medication may be needed at first to ensure that the patient has a regular bowel action, and the most natural type of laxative is a bulking agent such as Normacol or Celevac.

Dietary advice

1. Discover the patient's normal eating habits and his likes and dislikes.
2. Encourage him to drink at least two litres (eight glasses) of fluid daily.
3. Suggest how he can adapt his diet to include foods high in roughage – wholemeal bread instead of white bread; breakfast cereals such as Weetabix, All-Bran and Puffed Wheat should be encouraged and biscuits should be of the wholemeal variety (digestives).
4. Do not peel potatoes but wash and boil with the skin on. When cooking cabbage, include the stalks. Peas and beans have a relatively high fibre content. If possible, eat fruit raw and unpeeled.
5. Try two teaspoonfuls of unprocessed bran sprinkled on cereals, soups and sauces.

Other advice

1. Try and establish a regular time for defaecation – preferably after breakfast.
2. Do not ignore the initial urge to defaecate.
3. Flexion of the thighs on the abdomen helps to promote defaecation; placing a stool in front of the lavatory to support the feet assists in this flexion.
4. Take plenty of exercise (if fit enough) to improve the tone of the abdominal muscles.
5. Try and avoid drugs such as sedatives and codeine derivatives which are constipating.

When caring for the terminally ill the nurse must remember that analgesic drugs frequently cause constipation and so an aperient such as Dorbanex should be requested in conjunction with the analgesics.

CARE OF THE PATIENT WITH DIARRHOEA

Patients suffering from diarrhoea may be referred to the district nurse for help and advice. It helps if she understands the causes which may lead to this common and distressing symptom (Fig. 10/2). If the condition lasts for more than two or three days the patient should be examined by a general practitioner to elicit if possible, the cause. Talking to the patient and his family for the

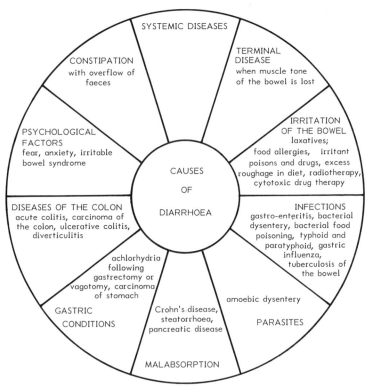

Fig. 10/2 Causes of diarrhoea

first time enables the district nurse to obtain a nursing history. Typical questions she should ask are:

1. How long has the patient been suffering from diarrhoea?
2. Has he ever had it before and, if so, what was the reason the doctor gave for the condition?
3. What are the patient's normal bowel habits?
4. How many times a day does the patient have to defaecate at present?
5. Is the patient taking any tablets? If so, what are they and how long has he been taking them?
6. Has the patient passed any blood with his motions?
7. Has he had any pain or vomiting?
8. Has he eaten any foods to which he is unaccustomed?
9. Has he ever been constipated over a prolonged period of time?
10. Has he any particular worries at the moment?

Advice and care

The district nurse should advise the patient to reduce the roughage and gas-producing foods in his diet. A bland diet is helpful for a few days until there is improvement. If the patient can manage oral fluids these should be encouraged to prevent dehydration. The importance of cleanliness must be emphasised; the patient's anal area and buttocks must be washed and dried well following defaecation. When caring for this type of patient the nurse must wear a disposable plastic apron and gloves. If the diarrhoea is caused by a systemic disease, especially a terminal illness, the nurse may have to visit daily or possibly several times a day. Drugs such as codeine phosphate or a kaolin mixture may be prescribed.

ULCERATIVE COLITIS

An exacerbation of ulcerative colitis generally means admission to hospital, especially if this is acute. Nursing at home is possible, providing conditions are right. Bedrest is necessary to reduce intestinal motility. The patient is often emaciated, so skin care and the prevention of pressure sores are very important. Regular turning and position changing are part of the caring programme, together with cleanliness of the buttocks and anal area. A barrier cream should be used. Pyrexia is common during acute attacks of the disease so a daily blanket bath and intermittent washing of face, hands and other areas affected by perspiration are necessary to keep the patient comfortable.

Medication

Sulphonamides are often given to combat infection together with anti-inflammatory agents such as corticosteroids and possibly iron and vitamin supplements for anaemia. A course of prednisolone retention enemata given at night may alleviate the condition. Sometimes it is possible to teach the patient or a relative how to give this enema, otherwise the district nurse will have to visit to administer it. Codeine phosphate, by tablet, may be given to help the diarrhoea. The nurse must advise the patient to drink at least 2½ litres of fluid a day to replace that lost through the diarrhoea, and to prevent any adverse effects upon kidney function. Diet should be one of low roughage, high protein and high calorie with added vitamins B and C.

The district nurse should liaise, where necessary, with the social worker to ensure that any social problems are dealt with. Worry can cause a relapse, and sympathetic care is very important in establishing confidence in the nurse's ability to deal with any physical or psychological needs. Once the condition has improved the patient should be encouraged to return to work and told of the importance of a nourishing diet with the avoidance of foods that irritate the colon. A plan can be worked out for a balance between work, rest and recreation; chilling, exhaustion and contact with anyone suffering from an infection such as influenza should be avoided because these could precipitate a relapse.

INCONTINENCE

The district nurse is involved with many patients who are incontinent. In the United Kingdom, urinary incontinence is a social disease for nearly two million people causing humiliation, social isolation and often outright rejection. It may debar a person from obtaining a place in a nursing home; incontinent patients are not encouraged to enter social services Part III accommodation for the elderly.

First visit

As in any first visit the procedure follows the same pattern (see

p. 10). With an incontinent patient the district nurse will need to know the following:

1. How long has the patient been troubled by incontinence?
2. Did it start suddenly, or gradually over a period of time?
3. Does the patient feel he needs to pass urine frequently during the day?
4. How often (approximately)?
5. Does he have to get up during the night to pass urine? If so, how many times?
6. Does he feel he must empty his bladder at once?
7. Does he get much warning of wanting to pass urine?
8. Does he ever have an accident?
9. Does he ever wet himself without being aware of doing so? Is this leakage a little or a lot?
10. Does it occur occasionally, or all the time?
11. Does the patient ever have a small leakage of urine when he coughs or sneezes?
12. To a female patient – how many pregnancies? Did she have a forceps delivery or any damage needing stitches following the birth?
13. Does the patient have a regular bowel action, or is he prone to constipation?
14. Does he ever wet the bed at night?

After tactfully discussing with the patient the actual incontinence problem, the nurse should assess any environmental factors which might aggravate the condition. For instance, are there adequate lavatory facilities near at hand? (This could mean lavatory, commode or urinal.) Does the patient use a walking aid? Is the accommodation on one level or is the lavatory upstairs (or downstairs)? Does the patient sleep in a bed which is too high, thus making it difficult for him to get up in a hurry? Does the patient need help from someone to reach the lavatory? Is the person disabled and unable to remove underclothes in time before micturition starts?

In addition there is a possibility that the patient may be constipated. The nurse should tactfully ask if she can carry out a rectal examination to eliminate faecal impaction as a possible cause of incontinence. Other routine examinations include urinalysis and culture of a midstream specimen of urine. The patient's doctor will decide whether an intravenous pyelogram, cystometry, cystogram and cystoscopy are justified. He will also examine the patient to determine whether the incontinence is due to an enlarged prostate gland, fibroids or weakness of the pelvic floor muscles – all of which can be corrected by surgical procedures.

Management of the incontinent patient

The aim of management is to enable the patient and his family to cope with this disability. In many cases a cure can be achieved, and in all patients the condition can be helped by professional advice.

Stress incontinence can be helped by instruction in carrying out pelvic floor exercises. Today, most women are taught these exercises after childbirth and, if they are properly carried out at the time, stress incontinence is much less likely to occur later. Thus, effective post-natal teaching is of paramount importance.

Pelvic floor exercises

These exercises, which will be taught initially by a physiotherapist, should be carried out conscientiously for at least three months. The patient must be told to *persevere* as improvement will be very gradual.

1. Instruct the patient to sit, stand or lie comfortably, without tensing the muscles of the buttocks, legs or abdomen, then pretend to control diarrhoea by tightening the ring of muscle around the anus. This should be repeated several times until the patient is sure that he has identified the area and is making the correct movement.
2. Tell the female patient to sit on the lavatory or commode and start to pass urine. While doing this she should attempt to stop the flow in midstream by tightening the muscles around the 'front passage'. This exercise should be repeated several times until she is sure of the movement and the sensation of applying conscious control.
3. Lastly teach her the following, whether standing, sitting or lying down: first tighten the anal muscles and then the 'front passage' muscles, then tighten both together before releasing them. This can be carried out at any time, whether in bed, standing or sitting.

Incontinence charts

In hospital it is easy to keep an incontinence chart, observe the patient and establish a pattern of micturition. In the home it is more difficult. There is the patient who lives alone and who could not be relied upon to keep a chart and visit the lavatory regularly, for him it needs an organised team effort of nurses, home helps and volunteers to carry this out. If the patient lives with relatives and one of them is at home all day to help the patient to the lavatory and to complete the chart then the nurse will be able to gain some idea as to the type of incontinence which is causing the condition.

With the elderly the difficulty is often one of urgency. If two-hourly visits to the lavatory are not sufficient to keep the patient dry, then hourly visits may be necessary at first even if the patient does not feel the need to pass urine. An alarm clock or kitchen timer can be set to ring hourly or two-hourly; if hourly visits to the lavatory are needed, bladder drill may be helpful.

Bladder drill

When passing urine the patient should try to stop the flow and then start again, as in pelvic floor exercises. After several attempts the patient should then try to 'hold on', waiting a little longer each time before recommencing micturition. In this way the time interval is gradually extended. Bladder drill is a positive and practical action which the patient can carry out himself.

Other advice

First ensure that toilet facilities are not too far away. Alternatively provide a commode, bedpan or urinal. The nurse must tell the patient not to cut down on his fluid intake but should advise him to drink more in the earlier part of the day. If diuretics are part of his medication, these too should be taken early in the day to avoid the possibility of night incontinence. Similarly, night sedation can impair awareness of the need to micturate and cause nocturia and enuresis. This should be discussed with the GP.

Constipation must be avoided and dietary advice (if possible accompanied by a diet sheet) given. Clothes should be worn which are easy to remove, such as a wrap over skirt and specially adapted trousers. For disabled patients, aids such as a raised lavatory seat and suitably placed grab rails can make sitting down and getting up from the lavatory easier. For the wheelchair patient who uses a commode, the height of each should be the same to facilitate the transfer. For the severe stroke patient there are two problems: (a) he may not recognise a urinal or know what to do with it. He must be shown repeatedly how to use it so that he can relearn the action; and (b) he may be aphasic and unable to communicate his bodily needs. In this case a system will have to be worked out such as the ringing of a hand-bell when the urge to pass urine is felt.

Intractable incontinence

If the patient's incontinence cannot be completely controlled, regular visits to the lavatory must continue but, in addition, some form of protection will be needed to keep him comfortable and independent. When deciding which form of protective aid is the most suitable the following factors should be taken into account:

1. The amount of leakage, and whether it occurs at night, by day or both
2. Whether the patient is relatively mobile or is bedfast or wheelchair bound
3. The age, physical and mental condition of the incontinent person.

Various body-worn appliances are designed for the male incontinent patient. They fit on to the penis, and urine drains into a bag which is strapped to the leg and concealed inside the trouser leg. For female patients there are as yet no suitable appliances which collect urine. Some doctors recommend the use of an indwelling catheter but often absorbent pads and protective pants are the solution preferred by the patient. Most health authorities provide certain makes of protective pants, padding and underpads to protect the bed.

Odour control

Odour occurs when urine and faeces are exposed to the air. If a patient uses absorbent pads for his incontinence, they should be wrapped in newspaper or a plastic bag and placed in a bucket with a lid. Wet or soiled clothing should be removed and left to soak in water until it can be laundered. A deodorant such as Nilodor can be obtained from the chemist.

Most local authorities provide an incontinence collection service for pads and other refuse, and in a few areas there is an incontinence laundry service. Ideally a minimum of two deliveries and collections a week is recommended, with an adequate supply of linen on loan if necessary.

Medication

Recently, doctors have found that the use of anticholinergic drugs such as emepronium bromide (Cetiprin) can help in the management of frequency due to functional change, the management of the uninhibited neurogenic bladder, the irritable bladder, and in some cases the easing of stress incontinence. This drug should be used in conjunction with regular bladder training.

Faecal incontinence

Faecal incontinence is not necessarily a problem of old age. Attention to possible causes and positive management can make control possible. The spurious diarrhoea of faecal impaction can be treated and following dietary advice and aperients should be capable of prevention. Persistent diarrhoea can be due to various causes and should be investigated by the doctor. Neurological causes such as spinal cord lesions and severe dementia result in a loss of sphincter control. Often the regular administration of suppositories will give a normal bowel action and prevent faeces leaking from an incompetent sphincter. The use of disposable pads and protective pants make physical management easier.

A recent report (1983) *Improving Services for the Incontinent Adult* based on a survey carried out by the Disabled Living Foundation and Age Concern, Greater London, recommended:

1. Careful assessment of the incontinent patient.
2. Training of staff to develop the necessary approach to incontinence.
3. An incontinence adviser in each health district.
4. Availability of hospital facilities to investigate, diagnose and treat incontinence.
5. Wide publicity of local incontinence services.
6. Health districts to review their incontinence laundry services.
7. A disposal and collection service for soiled pads to be provided and advertised.
8. Supplies officers to keep up-to-date with the range of equipment available and to have samples available.
9. Agreement between the health district and social services as to which equipment each should supply.

UTERINE PROLAPSE

Many patients who suffer from this condition are now treated surgically but the district nurse may need to visit those who are treated palliatively by the insertion of a pessary.

Clinical features of a prolapse include backache, frequency of micturition, a feeling of discomfort when the patient is standing, a 'bearing down' sensation, stress incontinence and difficulty in passing urine and defaecating. The insertion of a pessary is indicated if the patient does not want surgery and where the prolapse is amenable to pessary support. It is also for the patient who is not fit for surgery or who wishes to delay this.

The district nurse may visit patients with bladder, bowel and genital problems other than those specifically mentioned. A number of visits are made to patients who have been discharged early from hospital after hysterectomy, sterilisation, anterior and posterior repair, oophorectomy, and prostatectomy. She removes sutures, and is ready to give advice and support where needed. Patients tend to be sensitive about many of these personal problems, and the nurse must use a tactful approach to gain confidence and give maximum support.

BIBLIOGRAPHY

Action on Incontinence. Report of a Working Group (1983). King's Fund Project Paper, London.

Breckman, B. (ed) (1981). *Stoma Care: A Guide for Nurses, Doctors, and Other Health Care Workers*. Beaconsfield Publishers, Beaconsfield.

Browne, B. (1978). *Management for Incontinence*. Age Concern England, Sutton, Surrey.

Mandelstam, D. (ed) (1980). *Incontinence and Its Management*. Croom Helm, Ltd, London.

Stoma Care – A Team Approach (1981). Royal College of Nursing, London.

Chapter Eleven

PSYCHIATRIC ILLNESS
AND MENTAL HANDICAP

PSYCHIATRIC ILLNESS

In England five million people consult their general practitioner each year about a psychiatric (mental health) problem. This does not mean that each one has to be referred to a psychiatrist and his team, but it does appear that psychiatric illness is on the increase. All members of the primary health care team, including the district nurse, need to be able to recognise the early signs and symptoms of psychiatric illness (especially depression) so that treatment can be started without delay.

Factors in the early recognition of psychiatric illness or abnormality

Awareness of those at risk
Awareness of how psychiatric illness may manifest itself
Detection of signs of confusion or self-neglect
Observation of a child's behaviour at home and possible need for help from a clinical or educational psychologist
Calling in specialist services if the patient's mental condition shows signs of relapsing

Risk factors

The absence of stability, love and affection in a child's home background
Continuous parental strife, divorce or separation
Incorrectly chosen occupation, resulting in strain and stress
Too rigid or ill-judged moral or cultural standards, or rejection by a parent
Onset of puberty, pregnancy, menopause, late middle-age and retirement – milestones when the risk of psychiatric illness is higher

Vitamin deficiency and viral diseases; chronic disabling
   conditions and terminal illnesses (factors in depression)
Bereavement
Loss of job and reduced earnings owing to illness
Drugs such as the oral contraceptive pill
Personal disfigurements following an accident or a surgical
   operation such as a mastectomy

Unfortunately there is often still a stigma attached to 'mental'
illness and the psychiatrically ill do not receive the same amount of
sympathy and understanding as do those who are physically ill.
With both types of illness, however, early detection and treatment
are important in order to ensure a more worthwhile life for the
patient and his family. Nowadays, more such patients are
maintained at home with the help of new methods of treatment
such as drug therapy. Short periods in hospital and active
treatment in outpatient departments and day hospitals help these
people to cope with their illnesses.
   District nurses may visit homes where there is a psychiatrically
ill family member; or psychiatric illness may result from a stress
situation within the home. This is usually aggravated by
personality traits and heredity factors inherent in the individual.
The nurse must always be aware of the possibility that caring for a
sick relative at home can become a strain on the family. She should
identify such 'at risk' situations in her assessment and planning of
care, and seek to provide help, support and counselling to relieve
tensions and individual problems. Regular visiting by the nurse
should enable her to observe the effectiveness of her attempts to
help the patient and his caring family and deal with further
problems as they arise. She must also be aware that other factors
such as drugs and alcohol and toxins can produce symptoms of
psychiatric illness. A knowledge of manifestations of common
psychiatric illnesses is invaluable to the district nursing sister when
she is assessing the needs of her patient and his family and helps her
to plan the care needed.

PSYCHIATRIC DISORDERS

Acute anxiety state

Anxiety is a common neurotic reaction to stress or a threat. It is
often a fear of the unknown which gives rise to recognised physical

symptoms affecting all the body systems. What appears to be trivial to one person may be overwhelming to another. Symptoms may include palpitations, sweating, gasping respirations and dilated pupils. There may be a sense of impending death or doom. Overbreathing with consequent alkalosis due to loss of carbon dioxide may occur. Reassurance and sedation form the basis of treatment of such 'panic attacks'. Obviously any situation which precipitated the attack should be investigated.

Chronic anxiety state

In this case symptoms tend to wax and wane. The level of anxiety will fluctuate according to the amount of stress present and the district nurse may be able to assist in relieving this by calling in various agencies to help care for sick and disabled family members who are contributing to the strain on the family as a whole. The person with a chronic anxiety state may complain of fatigue, tension headaches, diarrhoea or constipation, frequency of micturition, insomnia or tremor. Anxious people are more sensitive to incoming stimuli and the resultant distractedness means that they may well complain of difficulty in concentration, forgetfulness, a muddled feeling or fear of dying or going insane.

Treatment includes elimination of physical causes for the symptoms experienced. Stress situations must be ameliorated. Tranquillisers may be prescribed for the anxiety and hypnotics if there is a sleep disturbance. Admission for a short period to a psychiatric hospital may help the patient to uncover the unconscious root of his difficulties. Group, marital or family therapy may help him to analyse his problems. A sympathetic yet firm approach to such a patient is necessary to help him face reality.

Reactive depression

Most of us feel depressed at some stage of our lives but we eventually manage to 'snap out of it'. This type of depression is known as reactive depression because there are precipitating stressful factors in our lives which are responsible for this behavioural response. It is one of the most common mental illnesses encountered by the district nurse. The individual himself is usually hypersensitive and anxious and has great difficulty in dealing with stressful situations. Although there is an accepted clinical picture in that there is a cause for the depression, the patient will blame others for his illness. He is anxious and sometimes resentful and complains of tiredness, lack of concentration and insomnia. He may well feel better in the morning and get worse as the day goes on. He looks weary and lethargic and finds life dull and unexciting. Misery is apparent in his facial expression and he is not interested in his appearance. He complains of anorexia, weight loss and constipation and may believe that he is dying of some incurable disease.

Reactive depression is helped by relieving the underlying cause. Usually the patient can be treated effectively by his general practitioner with antidepressant drugs but sessions with a psychiatrist may help him come to terms with his feelings. A positive approach by all concerned is needed to encourage him to take an interest in living and in his family, friends and social life.

Endogenous depression

This usually occurs in the absence of any environmental stress and a heredity factor may be present. There may be a history of recurrent attacks of mania. The depression is severe and the person is unable to react with a normal show of emotion to events around him. Delusions of guilt, persecution and hypochondriasis are common. Hallucinations may occur. Insomnia is not usually a problem but early morning waking is often experienced. The risk of suicide should always be considered.

Hospital admission is desirable for the severely depressed patient who cannot be safely managed at home. Antidepressant drugs form the basis of treatment. Endogenous depression responds well to electroconvulsive therapy. A bright and stimulating environment is essential and the patient is encouraged, but not forced, to join in ward activities. A positive and consistent approach to these patients is important.

Dementia

Senile dementia is discussed in Chapter 8. The district nurse is sure to meet patients suffering from both senile and pre-senile dementia. Characteristics of the conditions include a decline in intelligence, loss of memory, an inverted sleep rhythm, irritability, anxiety, agitation, delusions of being robbed or neglected and irresponsible behaviour. Eventually talk becomes a mere babble of words and the patient is unable to comprehend the simplest tasks or instructions. Care in the community is possible initially but much support from both the statutory and voluntary services is needed to relieve the strain on the family. Regular holiday admissions are important to give them a rest. Regular evaluation of the care given and a problem solving approach to care is essential. Eventually permanent hospitalisation may be the only answer for those requiring intensive and constant care with many precautions for their safety.

Organic psychoses

The fact that an organic condition may be responsible for disturbed cerebral function has already been mentioned. Psychotic symptoms such as confusion, disorientation, memory impairment and hallucinations may result. Systemic causes include infections, metabolic disturbances, endocrine disorders, deficiency diseases and drug or alcohol intoxication. Cerebral causes include infection together with trauma, a tumour, degeneration or epilepsy. Once the cause of the condition is discovered and treated the psychotic symptoms disappear. The district nurse in her initial assessment of the needs of the patient may well pick up clues which indicate the cause of the patient's confusion. A pyrexia might indicate an infection. A low temperature coupled with a slow pulse, obesity and a dislike of the cold might indicate myxoedema. A cache of bottles of tablets in the cupboard or by the bed could mean that drugs are the culprit. Certainly the smell of alcohol on the patient's breath would lead the nurse to suspect this as the possible underlying cause for the confusion. A history of falls could indicate that a sub-dural haematoma might have been sustained. Tumours might produce signs such as loss of vision, a weakness on one side of the body or headaches. Any suspicions of an organic condition must be communicated immediately to the patient's general practitioner.

Manic-depressive psychoses

This condition is typified by alternating states of mania and depression – swings in mood from elation to despair. In fact a crisis may precipitate the first attack of mania and further attacks may accompany stressful situations. The patient is usually a warm and friendly person and these traits become exaggerated with the illness. The person devises ambitious plans which are impossible to fulfil. He is constantly moving about and talking rapidly and loudly. Indoors he feels hemmed in and wants to go out. Alternatively he may feel that his clothes are irritating him so off they come! He does not have time for eating or drinking and so easily becomes dehydrated and undernourished. If prevented from doing what he wants, he may become irritable and aggressive. He may eventually become unpopular with his family who become irritated by his behaviour.

Treatment is aimed at providing the patient with rest and nutrition and to protect him from injury. Sedation is essential. He must be coaxed to eat. His surroundings must be quiet and tranquil and nursing in isolation may be necessary if he is very disturbed.

Schizophrenia

The onset of schizophrenia often occurs in the adolescent or young adult. About 45 per cent of psychiatric hospital beds are occupied by schizophrenics. The main features of the condition are disturbances of emotion, thought, perception and volition which result in abnormal behaviour. The schizophrenic lives in a fantasy world divorced from reality. He is usually a shy, introverted person who appears to be trying to escape from the stresses of reality. There is thought to be a heredity factor, due to a recessive gene, which may lead to the development of schizophrenia.

Four main types – simple, hebephrenic, catatonic and paranoid – exist, although a patient may portray more than one characteristic of the disease and not fit into any one category.

The person with *simple schizophrenia* may escape diagnosis for some time as the onset is insidious in a young individual. He slowly becomes more preoccupied and solitary. Ultimately he may withdraw completely from society, neglecting both his work and his appearance until only hospital care can help him.

Hebephrenic schizophrenia also occurs in young people but the onset is rapid with a period of withdrawal followed by a phase of wild excitement. Symptoms include thought disturbances, flattening of emotion and strange delusions and hallucinations. He may be able to live a normal lifestyle but relapses are common.

Catatonic schizophrenia is more common in young females, who suffer alternating periods of stupor and excitement. She may adopt strange postures and mannerisms and although apparently in a stupor she can often relate afterwards all that has happened around her. She may repeat what has been said to her and at times is completely mute.

Paranoid schizophrenia occurs in later life and is typified by delusions, suspicion and hallucinations of being persecuted. The patient behaves as if his delusions were true.

Nowadays, the emphasis is on community care for the mentally ill wherever possible and if the schizophrenic has a caring family to return to he may be able to attend a local day hospital for supervision of his treatment and medication. The other alternative is accommodation in a hostel for the psychiatrically ill or a half-way house. The introduction of long-acting phenothiazines such as Modecate injections now form the basis of treatment of schizophrenia. These should preferably be administered by a community psychiatric nurse who will monitor their effects. Group therapy is another important part of the treatment aimed at helping the patient to establish relationships. Some schizophrenics take up painting or music while others are given simple work to do. Anorexia nervosa and both drug and alcohol addiction are classified by the World Health Organization as psychiatric illnesses. The first is a *neurosis* as the individual is expressing her difficulties in coping with the stresses of everyday living by developing this condition. The whole personality is not involved and the neurosis is based on learnt behaviour. Drug and alcohol addiction are considered to be *psychoses* as the individuals are not aware that they are ill. For them reality becomes distorted and their behaviour becomes bizarre.

In recent years the hospital service has developed a specialist therapeutic team consisting of psychiatrists, psychiatric nurses, psychotherapists and psychiatric social workers who are on call to deal with a psychiatrically ill patient. Where these teams have been set up, consultation and liaison with the primary health care teams has considerably improved the care given to such patients.

THE COMMUNITY PSYCHIATRIC NURSE (CPN)

Over the past 20 years, most psychiatric hospitals have reduced their in-patient population considerably, many by 40–50 per cent. This has come about because of the discovery of effective neuroleptic drugs, many of which are disease specific. Social skills and psychological techniques have been developed as treatment agents, and the harmful effects of institutionalisation in a mental hospital have been highlighted. A nurse experienced in working with psychiatric patients is therefore in great demand.

The majority of community psychiatric nurses are hospital-based. They work usually on a full-time basis and are attached to the psychiatrist from whom they receive their referrals. A few schemes exist where a community psychiatric nurse is employed by the community nursing division and is attached full-time to the health centre. In some parts of the country the social services employ such nurses; and elsewhere dual appointments, both local authority and health service, exist. Some community psychiatric nurses specialise in the care of the elderly mentally infirm in the community. A general practitioner attachment scheme whereby four CPNs have been attached to primary health care teams in Oxfordshire is at present in operation. However, due to lack of staff, the CPN can only cover a certain area within which are contained many general practitioners and their teams.

Role and function

The role and function of the community psychiatric nurse may be described as follows:

- Use of nursing skills to assess and supervise the care of individuals' mental and physical states.
- Assessment of progress and co-ordination, administration and supervision of psychiatric treatment as prescribed by the responsible medical officer.
- Education of patients and their relatives into the effects and symptoms of mental illness and the aims of treatment.
- To give advice to patients and relatives on services available within the community.
- To give support to patients and relatives and to involve them where appropriate in the treatment programme.
- The establishment of rapid and flexible visiting patterns to obviate crisis in the community.
- To act as a link between the patient, the hospital and community services. Liaison with other professionals in hospital and primary health care teams.
- Education of the public and other professionals on mental health matters. Research and planning of the community psychiatric nursing services.

Most district nurses are presently not involved in caring for many psychiatrically ill or handicapped people but with the changing emphasis from hospital to community care this may well change. It is important that she should understand how psychiatric illness can manifest itself and remember the situations which may precipitate it. Although the district nurse may not be attached to a team which benefits from the presence of an attached CPN, she should be aware of how to contact her colleague for advice should the need arise.

MENTAL HANDICAP

There are approximately 450 000 mentally handicapped people in England, of whom 110 000 are severely handicapped and 340 000 mildly so. The aim of all health service workers is to prevent disease and handicap wherever possible and various measures can be taken to prevent mental handicap from occurring:

1. Genetic counselling after the birth of one handicapped child to identify potentially high risk parents.
2. Blood tests during pregnancy for alphafetoprotein, and amniocentesis at 16 weeks of pregnancy to detect Down's syndrome.
3. Immunisation of girls aged 10 to 14 against rubella, which can cause damage to the fetus if a mother contracts it during the first three months of pregnancy.
4. The use of anti-D immunoglobulin to prevent haemolytic disease of the newborn.
5. Screening to detect phenylketonuria within 6 to 14 days of birth. If the Guthrie test is positive, the baby must have a special diet to eliminate the production of poisonous phenylalanine metabolites which cause mental subnormality.
6. Expert care during labour to reduce the risk of asphyxia or brain damage to the baby.
7. Special care of low birthweight babies.

Like other disabled people, the mentally handicapped have medical, social, psychological and educational needs, and in providing for these, interdisciplinary teamwork is essential. The government's White Paper *Better Services for the Mentally Handicapped*, mentioned the following: 'a satisfactory environment whether at home or in residential accommodation; the avoidance of unnecessary segregation; the provision of education, training, and occupation to develop ability, support families and to achieve a measure of independence.' There is now a change in emphasis from residential to community care; to living in small groups and in hostels within the community.

Local authority social service departments provide the following:

(a) Social work support and counselling of parents. Until the age of 17 the social worker liaises with the educational authorities and parents over the care of the mentally handicapped. After this age they are the concern of the social services department.
(b) Adult training centres for those over 17 to work in sheltered workshops or some kind of chosen employment.
(c) Practical help such as home helps, day nurseries, laundry services and 'sitters-in' to give parents a rest.
(d) Occupational therapy centres for activities such as handicrafts, group activities and clubs.
(e) Facilities for small groups to live in a house or hostel.
(f) Short-term care for two to three weeks to enable the family to have a complete break from care.
(g) Organisation of holidays, outings and clubs.

District nursing involvement

The aim in caring for the mentally handicapped is a training system which enables as many as possible to fit in with society and achieve their highest potential. This includes the learning of social habits, caring for bodily needs and achieving a degree of independence. The Jay Report (1979) on the care of the mentally handicapped placed more emphasis on the need for training and social care which should be the responsibility of the social services departments, instead of specialist and community nursing care.

There should be a multidisciplinary approach to the assessment and management of the mentally handicapped. This is a life-long problem for the family, the cause of much stress to the parents and affecting other children in the family in various ways. Regular holiday breaks from caring are important. There is a need for more training centres for children and adults, together with the provision of sheltered workshops. The nurse must be able to support, guide and give practical help where this is required. She must also be on the look-out for signs of stress within the family and know what facilities are available in the locality to help relieve this. It is important that the handicapped person's basic needs are catered for. Bodily cleanliness and skin care are important if one is to be accepted by society. So too is oral and dental hygiene. There is a greater risk of contracting gingivitis if the drug phenytoin is being taken on a long-term basis. Blepharitis is more common in the mentally handicapped and so care of the eyes and eyelids is equally important as a preventive measure. Finger- and toenails should be kept sort and clean. A well-balanced diet should be provided and should contain plenty of roughage to prevent the development of constipation. Most mothers discover their own particular remedy for this. Bladder and bowel training is another important step towards achieving socialisation. Some severely handicapped patients are doubly incontinent and require plastic pants, padding, incontinence sheets and mackintosh sheets. Some need help in and out of the bath. If the patient has a persistent nasal or aural discharge the nurse should consider the possibility that a foreign body is present in the meatus. Above all else a safe environment in which to live is of most importance to the mentally handicapped, who are inquisitive and do not understand what may be dangerous for them to touch or in play. The district nurse should be on the look-out for obvious home hazards.

Mentally handicapped individuals can fall physically ill and so need the care provided by the district nursing service. Because the patient's level of understanding is subnormal the district nurse's approach must be sensibly adjusted. Simple explanations and demonstrations may be needed to gain the patient's co-operation. A friendly approach is essential.

General features of mental handicap

Abnormal physical features

Inability to think or formulate ideas adequately

Short attention span, easily distracted and subsequent learning difficulties

Behavious disorders such as aggression, hyperactivity, awkwardness, destructiveness, mannerisms, head-banging and rocking movements

Social learning is slow because they do not learn from past experiences so as to foresee the results of their actions

There may be associated physical and emotional conditions such as epilepsy, congenital heart disease and cerebral palsy.

Special aspects of care

It is important that the mentally handicapped person develops those abilities that he possesses. Exercises are needed to aid physical development which is slowed down in the mentally handicapped. Sitting and walking are delayed and muscle coordination is poor. This is where the physiotherapist and remedial gymnast can do much to help.

The individual's psychological needs are met by ensuring that the environmental atmosphere is warm, friendly and secure. A positive approach using praise rather than blame should be used to provide motivation to persevere. Consistency is also important. Behaviour modification is used to help the person achieve the desired behaviour, and positive reinforcement in the form of rewards is normally used.

The person suffering from cerebral palsy will have muscular disabilities due to brain damage or impaired development. Management in this case aims to prevent deformity with the use of appliances and possible surgical operations. The epileptic must take his medication regularly to ensure adequate blood levels of his anticonvulsants, and observation of the effects and side-effects of the drugs is needed. The hyperactive person needs constant observation to prevent him from harming himself. Soothing music and sedatives may help. There is often a reason for a mentally handicapped person to become aggressive. The main thing is to discover the cause and then modify the management of the person accordingly.

Mental handicap is a multi-faceted problem needing cooperation and participation by a multidisciplinary team.

REFERENCES

DHSS (1970). *Better Services for the Mentally Handicapped*. Cmnd. 4683. HMSO, London.
Report of the Committee of Enquiry into Mental Handicap Nursing and Care (the Jay Report) (1979). HMSO, London.

BIBLIOGRAPHY

Clarke, D. (1982). *Mentally Handicapped People. Living and Learning*. Baillière Tindall, London.
Malin, N., Race, D. and Jones, G. (1980). *Services for the Mentally Handicapped in Britain*. Croom Helm Ltd, London.

Chapter Twelve

CHILD HEALTH

CHILD HEALTH IN THE COMMUNITY

Preventive health services for children are part of the health visitor's work, and during the first days of a baby's life the midwife is also involved. Preventive services include:

Help in avoidance of prematurity
In some areas, the care of a premature baby at home by the domiciliary premature baby service
Advice and help with infant feeding
Child health clinics
The follow-up of children in 'at-risk' groups
Checking the normal stages of development
Advice about the safety of young children
Visiting a child in his home
Support and advice for parents with handicapped children
Care of acute illness in the one-to-five-year age-group.

SCHOOL HEALTH SERVICES

The school health service cares for children from the age of five years onward with the child's general practitioner. Emphasis is placed on the early diagnosis of disabilities to allow for correction and treatment. The service is also involved in the promotion of positive health and the arrangement of the educational programme for various groups of handicapped children. The health surveillance includes routine medical inspections, hygiene advice, the investigation of communicable diseases, health education, immunisations, preventive dental treatment, school clinics and cleanliness inspections.

When parents do not bring their young children to the child health clinic for regular health and developmental checks and immunisations, it is the duty of the health visitor to follow up this non-attendance and discuss what might be done. In some districts the district nurse runs immunisation clinics in conjunction with the health visitor and in other areas a clinic nurse is employed by the health authority specifically for this purpose. Child immunisation is generally regarded as an 'extended role' task and extra training is needed and a proficiency certificate awarded.

FACTORS AFFECTING CHILD HEALTH

The whole structure of society is changing and the growing child is part of this change. The age of marriage is falling and young adults have no chance of following the example of their parents and acquiring the skills associated with parenthood. Families are smaller so older children no longer care for younger brothers and sisters. Child-rearing patterns have changed and increasingly both parents work – thus giving rise to the problem of who is to care for the children. Young couples move away from their family town to seek employment, so there are no relatives to help out. The divorce rate nationally is in the range of one in every three marriages; this causes breakdown in normal family life and the stress involved is bound to affect the child. Many children are members of a one-parent family, which often creates a lower standard of living; and an increasing number of children are now seen by child psychiatrists and educational psychologists because of behavioural and learning problems.

The main cause of death in the four-to-five-year age-group is accident in the home, followed by road traffic accident. At least one child will die each year from battering. With the advent of prophylaxis, the death rate from infectious diseases has fallen dramatically but parents have become complacent and are unaware of the danger if immunisation is neglected. Some areas are more deprived than others; high infant and neonatal mortality rates led to the setting-up of the Court commission. The Court Report (*The Future of the Child Health Services*) was published in 1976 and suggested the introduction of a total paediatric specialisation within existing primary health services. In the report it was hoped that a child health visitor (CHV) might be appointed with both curative and preventive nursing responsibilities. Under her direction child health nurses (CHNs) would teach parents how to prepare infant feeds and care for sick children at home. In many ways it endorsed the recommendations of the Platt Report (*The Welfare of Children in Hospital*) with regard to the need for paediatric community sisters so that ill children can be nursed where possible at home. In some urban areas now there are paediatric home nursing schemes and a large proportion of their work is in caring for children who have had day case surgery.

DAY CASE SURGERY

Many children are now operated on as day cases for two reasons: (a) it is undesirable to separate a young child from his mother unless this is absolutely essential; and (b) if the child is admitted to hospital for one day only, more hospital beds are available for others needing surgery.

The child and his mother are seen by the consultant in the outpatient department. If operative treatment is necessary the mother will be given the approximate date of admission, in order that she may organise the rest of her family and stay in the hospital with the child that day. Sometimes the health visitor or nursing sister may be asked to visit the family at home to assess the child's social and domestic background before the decision is taken to treat the child as a day case.

The parents are sent a form with instructions that the child must not be given any food or drink from midnight the night before his admission. Because of the importance of this instruction, full explanation of the reason for it should be included.

The child is taken to hospital at 8 a.m. and the operation takes place during the following morning, after which he is allowed to recover from the anaesthetic and an ambulance takes him home, from 4 p.m. onward. The mother is asked to put the child to bed, and he will probably sleep through until the next morning. The district nurse (or paediatric sister) will have discussed with the ward sister which children are having operations, and will then visit each home that evening, or on the following day. She will give nursing advice where necessary and continue to visit until the child has recovered. The mother should know to whom she can telephone in case of need.

The following operations may be carried out on a day case basis: circumcision, herniorrhaphy, orchidopexy, minor orthopaedic procedures and investigation of bladder and bowel function. The use of absorbable suture material by some surgeons has abolished the need for suture removal.

THE SICK CHILD AT HOME

A sick child nursed at home will be less apprehensive than one admitted to a hospital ward. If he is old enough, any procedures should be explained to him by the district nurse (the use of a favourite toy will help at such times). When nursing a sick child, as many activities as possible should be turned into play. An ill child who is happily occupied is likely to recover more quickly than one who is not so. A child can appear to be desperately ill, and an hour or two later is sitting up and playing.

One of the original reasons for the provision of district nurses was to care for children suffering from infectious diseases. Nowadays, with the use of antibiotics and prophylaxis, childhood infections are less severe and rarely need trained nursing, but the district nurse may be asked by a worried mother for advice on how to care for a child with an infectious disease or other childhood problems, so she must keep herself up-to-date with current advice and practice.

Worms

Advice is often sought if worms are suspected. The tiny *threadworm* or larger *roundworm* can be seen excreted in the lavatory. In the former case there is intense irritation in the anal area. Sleeplessness and irritability are common. The child with roundworm infestation has few signs and symptoms other than the presence of worms in the faeces. Piperazine sulphate and senna (Pripsen) is the treatment of choice. One single dose is given, followed by a second dose after 7 to 10 days. All members of the family should be treated.

The sight of a length of *tapeworm* in the faeces is alarming to parents and they need reassurance that the infestation will respond to treatment. This consists of an oral dose of dichlorophen with a drink before breakfast on two successive mornings. The drug destroys the worm and it is digested in the bowel before the aperient action of the dose takes effect.

Lice and nits

The head louse reproduces by means of hatching eggs which are attached to the hair follicles with a 'cement-like' substance. This makes removal of the eggs (nits) difficult. Treatment is by shampooing the hair with a pesticidal and ovicidal shampoo such as Derbac. A fine-toothed comb should be used afterwards to remove the nits. The shampooing should be repeated after eight days and the whole family must be treated.

Gastro-enteritis

Gastro-enteritis in babies can lead rapidly to dehydration which necessitates admission to hospital. The child nursed at home should not be given any food for at least 24 hours. Plenty of clear fluids should be encouraged with a pinch of salt being added to each glass, disguised by the addition of fruit juice. The doctor may prescribe a kaolin mixture to 'settle' the gastro-intestinal tract. When the child has not vomited or had diarrhoea for 24 hours he can be given drinks of half-strength milk and, if all is well, a light, easily-digested diet can be slowly introduced and the child gradually returned to normal meals.

Soiled garments and bedding should be thoroughly washed and sterilised, if possible by boiling.

Respiratory conditions

Acute bronchitis

Acute bronchitis is a condition which frequently attacks children from overcrowded homes, who are undernourished and debilitated. It is a common complication of measles, influenza, fibrocystic disease of the pancreas, congenital heart disease and Down's syndrome.

The mother should be advised to nurse the child in a warm, well-ventilated room, supported in bed with plenty of pillows. Clothing should be light but warm. The child and his mother should be aware of the need to change his position in bed at regular intervals – this moves the secretions in the air passages and prevents the formation of mucous plugs. Fluids are to be encouraged, and in particular warm drinks such as milk and honey, which will help relieve an irritating cough. The doctor may prescribe antibiotics to combat infection.

Bronchiectasis

This condition can result from the blockage of a bronchus, or following whooping cough or measles. The child is pale, undernourished and underdeveloped. He often suffers from respiratory-tract infections, otitis media and a chronic cough. The sputum is green and purulent, and, if swallowed, causes gastric irritation and loss of appetite. The child's schooling will be interrupted by repeated infections and illnesses.

The nurse can reinforce the teaching of the physiotherapist by supervising breathing exercises and ensuring that both the patient and parents are aware of the need to carry out postural drainage at least twice a day. Expectoration must be encouraged. A warm drink first thing in the morning helps this, together with inhalations and the instillation of nose drops to help loosen the secretions. Plenty of paper tissues should be available for the child's use and these, together with disposable sputum containers, should be put in a paper bag and wrapped in newspaper before being placed in the dustbin. The tissues can be burnt if an open fire or solid fuel boiler is available. Fresh air and exercise are to be encouraged and a nutritious diet with an increased protein content provided for the child.

Asthma

The asthmatic child is pale and underweight with a poor posture. A slight expiratory wheeze is usually apparent due to a constant mild degree of bronchial spasm. Such a child is often intelligent but very highly strung and nervy. The parents may be over-protective and in some cases emotional disturbances in the home can contribute to an exacerbation of the condition.

Management includes the avoidance of factors which precipitate asthmatic attacks. The child's bedroom should be warm, dry and well-ventilated. The aim is to eliminate dust mites and dry scales from bedding and its surroundings. A synthetic mattress and pillows are best and the former should be vacuum-cleaned at least once a week. If the presence of animals tends to provoke asthmatic attacks, it may fall to the nurse to explain that they will need to be removed from the household. During an acute attack of asthma, admission to hospital may become necessary, and the mother will be taught postural drainage and percussion so that she can clear excess mucus from the child's airways. The district nurse will encourage the mother to continue this treatment when the child returns home.

The most commonly used drug for the treatment and relief of asthma in a child is sodium cromoglycate (Intal) and it is administered through an inhaler. Children as young as four years can be taught to use it. Asthma can be exercise-induced, but if the child inhales Intal a few minutes before exercise the protection against an asthmatic attack will last for about an hour. Steroids are given only if attacks are frequent and severe.

Acute rheumatism

This disease is rare due to the reduced virulence of the causative agent (the group A beta-haemolytic streptococcus) and because of improved living standards. The condition follows one to four weeks after a streptococcal respiratory-tract infection and the child can be nursed at home if no complications are apparent. The treatment consists of bedrest, oral penicillin and salicylates. Careful observation of the child by the nurse for signs of salicylate overdose (nausea, tinnitus, vomiting, deafness, proteinuria, rashes) is essential and she will also watch for any complications. These include cardiac involvement, which is heralded by irregularities of the pulse rate and rhythm. A daily sleeping pulse rate should also be recorded. The mother must keep a fluid balance chart so that any imbalance between intake and output may be recorded, as this could be the beginning of cardiac failure. The nurse will need to visit several times a day. Caring for the child is a great strain on the mother, who must assist the child in all things to prevent exertion, and if there are other children in the family, admission to hospital may be considered necessary. The child's need to be kept amused and occupied during this lengthy illness is an added factor.

Juvenile rheumatoid arthritis (Still's disease)

The usual age for the onset of this disease is eighteen months to six years – the earlier the onset, the less favourable the prognosis. The condition appears abruptly and starts with a high fever and generalised joint pains; deformities occur due to bony growth disturbances and muscle wasting; thus there is a retardation of normal physical development. The course of the disease is characterised by relapses and remissions, and with each relapse more deformities.

Treatment consists of bedrest to relieve the strain on the weight-bearing joints and reduce pain.

The child lies on a sheepskin to prevent pressure sores developing, with light bedclothes supported by a bedcradle to prevent pressure on painful joints. Pillows, sandbags and splinting of painful limbs are required to prevent deformity. All joints are put through a full range of movement every 24 hours.

The child should be given a nutritious diet with added vitamins and including fresh fruit to prevent constipation. Suitable analgesia will be prescribed for joint pains. Iron tablets may be needed to combat anaemia.

The child's morale and interest must be maintained by continuing as much as possible with schoolwork and providing various occupations to amuse him.

At least 50 per cent of children who have this disease will recover with no residual joint lesions. The emphasis is on early diagnosis and treatment. Inadequate or late treatment may result in generalised ill-health, retarded growth, limb deformities and iridocyclitis which could result in blindness. Both acute rheumatism and Still's disease are now rarely seen by district nurses.

Leukaemia

The treatment of leukaemia in childhood usually consists of steroids and cytotoxic drugs to gain a remission or a cure. The leukaemic child is often very ill and much care is needed to keep him comfortable. The district nurse and the child's mother together undertake daily personal hygiene procedures and great care has to be taken while lifting the child to prevent bruising. The teeth are cleaned with cotton-wool swabs to avoid gum damage. Further mouth care includes regular mouthwashes, the application of petroleum jelly to prevent cracked lips, oral nystatin if thrush is present, and the application of gentian violet to any mouth ulcers. If the child has an epistaxis the mother should be shown how to apply ice to the bridge of the nose, and if this is ineffective she should be warned to contact the doctor.

There are no dietary restrictions, but the child should drink plenty of fluids, be given added vitamins and if possible eat fresh fruit to prevent constipation. An aperient may be needed if the child has a sore mouth and cannot eat foods with a high roughage content. Analgesics can be given to ease painful joints and induce rest and sleep.

Cytotoxic drugs have many side-effects. The child's resistance to infection is lowered. His room should be light and airy, and no one with an infection should approach him. Some drugs cause alopecia or thinning of the hair. A mild baby shampoo should be used and the hair tidied with a soft brush. Suitable wigs can be obtained through the National Health Service as baldness is distressing to both child and parents.

When the leukaemic child is being nursed at home it is often the mother and close family who do most of the caring. The district nurse visits daily, or more frequently if necessary, but often her role is more of a supporter of the carers. She teaches them how to look after their sick child and reassures them that they are doing it correctly. She deals with problems as they arise and liaises with her health visitor and social worker colleagues to ensure that the family get every support. She will keep the general practitioner informed of changes in the child's condition, and seek his help if problems arise.

Spina bifida

A child with spina bifida will encounter problems affecting the activities of daily living; walking difficulties, wasting of the legs, deformities of the feet and sphincter disturbances, such as incontinence. A spina bifida child will never have known normality or been aware of posture, sensation or balance, and the aim is to incorporate the child into a normal social environment.

The stress associated with giving birth to a child with spina bifida can lead to neglect or over-protection. The nurse is involved in teaching parents how to care for their child. All should be aware of the danger of trophic ulceration developing because of skin anaesthesia. Daily checks should be made for signs of redness and discolouration. The position in bed should be varied so that he is not always lying in the same place. He should be taught to lift himself off his buttocks every hour for at least 20 seconds if he is in a wheelchair. The skin should be washed each time any incontinence padding is changed, dried thoroughly and a barrier cream applied.

Urinary problems may range from stress incontinence to a complete loss of sphincter control. The child may get an over-distended bladder with the consequent risk of infection and need for antibiotics. The nurse must teach the mother (and later the child) how to express this urine manually if the bladder does become over-distended, and the child should be placed on a specially designed commode for this procedure.

Bowel management is less problematic, and generally

continence can be maintained by giving the child a diet low in roughage and a disposable enema once or twice a week. The nurse will show the mother how to carry out this procedure. Some children with spina bifida can achieve voluntary defaecation by straining at stool following a hot drink or a meal.

The occupational therapist will arrange for the necessary equipment to be installed in the home to assist in the care of the child. An open polyester foam mattress which is washable should be placed on the bed – no rubber or plastic should be used in order to prevent maceration. A plastic sling seat with a metal frame can be used when bathing to provide support and ensure safety. The physiotherapy department under the direction of an orthopaedic consultant will supervise the child's rehabilitation and provide the necessary walking aids. Orthoses may be fitted and will need to be assessed regularly by the orthotist. Hydrotherapy facilities may be available. It is hoped that the child can be sufficiently mobilised to avoid a wheelchair life but for some this is inevitable.

If a child also has hydrocephalus which is treated with a Spitz-Holter (or other) valve, then the mother must be taught to 'milk' the valve tube once or twice a day to prevent it from blocking.

The parents of a handicapped child will need much support. The district nurse will help with any practical procedures, and the health visitor will visit the family regularly throughout the child's life to offer advice and support.

The dying child

Once active treatment has ceased the dying child can be nursed at home if this is the wish of the parents, but they may feel better able to cope if the child is in hospital. Obviously they will feel more confident if their child is in hospital where professional help is always at hand, so if the child is being cared for at home it is vital that he is visited regularly by both the GP and community nursing staff. Visits should be increased as the condition deteriorates and parents should be given telephone numbers whereby they can contact the doctor or nurse at any time should the need arise.

It is important that the district nurse should be involved in the care of the terminally ill child long before the terminal stage arrives. In this way she can form a relationship with both the child and his family which will be invaluable later on. If she is only called in during the last week of life the child will not know or trust her and the parents will not be able to talk to her and share their grief.

An assessment of both the needs of the child and those of his family should be made on the initial visit and these must be reviewed regularly to ensure that the child is comfortable and the family is not under too much of a strain and can cope with all that is involved. It is important that the child should be allowed to lead as normal a life as possible within his capabilities. The caring team, especially the parents, should try to maintain his interests and give him something to strive for, a target to reach or a goal to achieve.

The child's response to his illness

Various factors affect this, including the child's age and level of development, pain, the type of symptoms, the type of treatment, the resultant changes in his lifestyle, and the attitudes and behaviour of others. The child who is becoming independent may be frustrated because he is deprived of that freedom by illness and is dependent on his parents again. Infants to a certain extent do not fare too badly if cared for at home but tend to be disturbed by a strange environment and separation from their mothers. School-age children may be limited in what they can do and become bored. This is where school work should be purposeful, occupational therapy creative and hobbies adapted to the child's physical ability.

It is important when caring for an older child to be sensitive to his fears and aspirations. Allow him to talk about his illness. He may well sense the severity of his condition. Parents themselves may convey their own anxiety to the child when distressed by his symptoms. Pain is more specific in an older child. He may react with rage and resentment against his parents and anyone looking after him. It is vital that this pain is dealt with adequately because no child should suffer unnecessarily nor should the trusting relationship between child, parents and nurses be weakened.

Treatment is accepted best in infancy as then it becomes part of the daily routine. Older children dislike it because it is a symbol of the illness and makes them different from their pals. Careful explanations should be given as to the nature and usefulness of the required regime – it is not a punishment. There is always the danger that parents may become over-zealous in carrying out the therapy and nursing care yet neglect the child's emotional and intellectual needs. This child is likely to become over-dependent on his parents. On the other hand the sick child may protest against his therapy. The parents must be warned to be firm when giving treatment as the child will exploit any signs of weakness.

Parental attitudes

In a way the parents suffer a double bereavement, first when told the diagnosis and second when the child actually dies. There may be a long interval in between. On being told of their child's diagnosis the initial reaction is one of shock and disbelief – this can't happen to me! They may ask for a second opinion and this should not be denied them. Once they have accepted the reality of their child's illness they will have many questions to ask. These must be answered truthfully so that they understand the situation. It is common to find parents blaming themselves for their child's illness and they need reassurance that there is nothing that they could have done to avert this and that they have done nothing to cause it. Alternatively they may direct the blame on others. Their aggression may cover their own feelings of guilt. At this stage it is better to direct their energies towards caring for the child. The district nurse should allow them to do as much of the actual caring for the child as possible. This is therapeutic in that they will always know that they did everything they could and have nothing to blame themselves for. Most firms are sympathetic and will allow the father time off from work, or more suitable working hours.

Care of siblings

Children are often more resilient than adults. If they ask if their brother or sister is dying, it is better to be optimistic initially but less so towards the end. Attention seeking behaviour is common among siblings of a terminally ill child. It might be a good idea to try and involve the other children in the caring process, praising and even rewarding them occasionally for all the help given. A sympathetic relative or friend may be able to help fill the gap left by the parents at this sad time.

Nursing the terminally ill child at home is not physically demanding as he will be light-weight, easily moved and pressure sores are rare if he is lying on a sheepskin. Incontinence is easy to manage with the use of drawsheets and incontinence pads but the child should still be sat on a 'potty' or commode regularly until he is too weak. Pain is treated with paracetamol or stronger analgesics if necessary and the effectiveness of the medication is constantly monitored by the nurse and parents. In conditions such as leukaemia and respiratory failure, which are distressing, diamorphine may have to be given in large doses, by injection if necessary.

The role of the district nurse is to demonstrate to the parents how to care for their sick child and make him comfortable. She constantly assesses the changing needs of both the child and his family and seeks to relieve problems as they arise. She co-ordinates the involvement of other agencies and reports back to the general practitioner any changes in the child's condition. Most important of all, the district nurse gives support to the parents and helps them to live through their grief. She may well visit them, as a friend who has shared that sad time with them, for some time after the child has died.

REFERENCES

The Future of the Child Health Services (Court Report) (1976). HMSO, London.
The Welfare of Children in Hospital (Platt Report) (1959). HMSO, London.

BIBLIOGRAPHY

Gyulay, J. E. (1978). *The Dying Child.* McGraw-Hill Book Co Ltd, Maidenhead.
McCarthy, G. T. (ed) (1984). *The Physically Handicapped Child: An Interdisciplinary Approach to Management.* Faber and Faber, London.
Woods, G. E. J. (1983). *Handicapped Children in the Community.* John Wright and Sons Limited, Bristol.

CLINICAL PROCEDURES AND EMERGENCY CARE

District nurses are 'generalists'. They have to adapt their skills to the situation in which they find themselves. They have to ensure that they are safe practitioners of nursing care, no matter what the setting. Obviously the majority of their work does occur in the patient's home – be this high-rise city flat or isolated country cottage with no mains water or drainage. It might be a residential home for the elderly run by the social services department or a private rest home.

Some nursing procedures may be carried out in the health centre or doctor's surgery where the district nurse runs a clinic session. District nurses (unlike practice nurses) are employed by the district health authority to whom they are responsible administratively. Only clinically are they responsible to the general practitioner. It is important that the district nurse only carries out procedures in which she is thoroughly competent and the employing authority and her senior nurse should know and approve of the arrangement. Some, such as venepuncture and immunisations, are classed as extended role tasks by many health authorities and instruction and regular up-dating has to be provided, but the district nurse is responsible for her own actions, and she should, therefore, belong to a professional organisation which provides legal protection. (Immunisations will not be discussed further.)

Some health authorities have their own procedure handbooks for their district nurses. This section is aimed at helping district nurses who work in health districts which do not have formal written procedures. It is also useful for practical work teachers who have to teach district nursing students how to carry out various procedures which they may not have had the opportunity to practise during their general training. It is an opportunity for all district nurses to examine their own practice.

FIRST AID FOR ANAPHYLACTIC SHOCK

Fortunately anaphylactic shock, characterised by severe bronchospasm, laryngeal oedema, urticaria and collapse, is extremely rare. However, it is obvious that those who administer drugs that may cause anaphylactic shock ought to be capable of diagnosing and treating this emergency correctly and adequately.

Most cases are caused by injections of drugs and the most hazardous in this respect are the penicillins and cephalosporins; streptomycin; vaccines, toxoids and antisera; and the hormones, adrenocorticotrophin (ACTH) and tetracosactrin.

The district nurse *must* ensure she knows the local policy for the administration of the above drugs and for dealing with the emergency of anaphylaxis. Ideally, community nurses should receive special lectures and written instructions on the diagnosis and treatment of anaphylactic shock and should be authorised to administer drug treatment on their own initiative. One recommended course of first aid actions is:

1. Lie the patient down and loosen any tight clothing about the neck.
2. Give adrenaline 1:1000 solution 0.5ml by intramuscular injection as soon as possible – reduce the dose in the elderly or those of slight build.

    Children up to 1 year – give 0.05ml; 1 to 5 years – give 0.1–0.4ml; 6 to 12 years – give 0.5ml.
3. Call for medical assistance if no one was available to do so earlier.
4. Repeat the dose after 10 minutes if no significant improvement has occurred, and again after 30 minutes if the patient's condition remains a cause for concern.
5. The nurse must renew her supply of adrenaline ampoules at specified intervals so that she is always prepared to deal with such an emergency. Discoloured ampoules should be replaced immediately.

PROCEDURES INVOLVING THE EYE

1. In all eye treatment use an aseptic technique.
2. Be gentle and precise in all movements.
3. In cases of infection or inflammation, care for the unaffected eye first.

4. Avoid touching the cornea as this is the most sensitive part of the eye.
5. Check carefully any preparation – correct patient, correct drug, correct eye, correct time, not out of date, correct amount.
6. Ascertain if the ointment is to be placed in the conjunctival sac or applied to the lid margins.

Instillation of eye drops/ointment

Equipment

Eye drops or ointment
Paper tissues

Method

1. Sit patient comfortably with head tilted backward or else lie the patient on a couch.
2. Explain procedure.
3. Wash hands.
4. Stand behind the patient and draw the lower lid downward.
5. With the pipette held 3cm above the eye allow the prescribed number of drops to fall into the lower fornix, not directly on to the cornea.
6. Tell the patient to close his eyes, then blink two or three times.
7. Wipe lashes once with a paper tissue.
8. Place an eye pad over the eye if this is ordered – ensure the patient closes his eye before doing this. Secure with tape.

Eye ointment is dispensed either in single-dose containers (Aplicaps) or in multidose tubes.

1. Pull the lower lid downward in the same way and squeeze a thin line of ointment into the lower fornix.
2. Tell the patient to close his eye.
3. Wipe excess ointment away with a tissue.
4. Warn the patient his vision may be blurred for a few minutes.

Irrigation of the eye

This is usually carried out to remove excess discharge from the eye, or as a first aid measure to remove foreign bodies or chemicals.

Equipment

Cape or towel
Tissues

Lotion thermometer
Receiver
Undine
Irrigating solution as ordered by the doctor. Examples include:
    Normal saline
    Sodium bicarbonate for acid burns ⎫
    Boracic acid for alkaline burns   ⎬ at 37°C
    Eye drops if ordered   ⎭

Method

1. The best position is for the patient to lie supine on a couch; alternatively he can sit in a chair and tip his head backward.
2. Protect his chest and shoulders with a cape or towel.
3. Prepare the equipment on a protected near-by table.
4. Fill the undine with the solution at the correct temperature.
5. Ask the patient (or a relative) to hold the receiver under the eye close to the cheek and to tilt his head to allow the solution to run into the receiver.
6. Stand behind the patient – if irrigating the left eye, hold the undine in the right hand, and vice versa.
7. Hold the undine about 4cm from the eye and direct the flow from the nasal to the temporal side.
8. First, tell the patient to look downward while you irrigate the eye and lift the upper lid against the upper margin of the orbit.
9. Second, instruct him to look upward as you depress the lower lid against the lower margin of the orbit, and irrigate the eye again.
10. Dry gently with soft tissues.
11. Insert drops or ointment as ordered by the doctor.
12. Cover with eye pad if requested.

Removal and care of artificial eyes

Equipment

Basic dressing pack
A second galipot
Normal saline solution at 37°C
Either, a glass rod (check it is not chipped) or sterile disposable gloves

Method

1. To remove the artificial eye, ask the patient to look up.

2. Press finger against upper eyelid and gently insert glass rod or gloved finger under the lower edge of the artificial eye, having pulled down the lower eyelid.
3. Grasp the lower edge of the artificial eye in the fingers of the right hand (being careful not to scratch or pinch the conjunctiva of the lower lid).
4. Place artificial eye in the second galipot.
5. Bathe the eyelid and note any discharge present.
6. Instil eye drops or apply ointment to the socket, if prescribed.
7. Carefully wash the artificial eye in normal saline, taking care not to scratch or chip it.
8. Re-insert the eye by asking the patient to look up, insert the eye under the upper eyelid, pull down the lower eyelid and gently press lower edge into position.

Important: Make certain that the notch of the artificial eye is at the top on the nasal side of the socket.

PROCEDURES INVOLVING THE EAR AND HEARING
Instillation of ear drops

Reasons

1. To soften the wax, using glycerine or Cerumol drops.
2. To treat otitis externa.

Method

1. Ask the patient either to lie down with the auditory meatus facing upward, or to sit and tilt the head sideways.
2. Warm the oily drops, but not the antibiotic ones.
3. If no applicator is supplied a warm teaspoon can be used to insert the prescribed number of drops.
4. Remove any excess drops with a tissue.
5. Ask patient to remain in this position for a few minutes.
6. Plug the ear with a small piece of cotton wool coated with white petroleum jelly, to prevent absorption of the drops.

Insertion of wick into the ear

Reasons

1. To treat localised external otitis due to infection.
2. To treat other types of otitis.

Equipment

Ribbon gauze for the wick
Sterile scissors
Sterile Tilley aural forceps
Galipot for the medicament
(Bacteriological swab and request form if required)
Disposable gloves

Method

1. Remove excess discharge using a tissue – take the swab now if required.
2. Wash your hands and put on the disposable gloves.
3. Cut off 4–6cm of ribbon gauze and soak in the medicament in the galipot.
4. Gently insert the wick into the external auditory meatus using the sterile aural forceps.
5. Cut off excess ribbon gauze.
6. Tell the patient to leave it in place for the required time but contact his doctor if his ear condition worsens.

Ear syringing

Reasons

1. Removal of foreign bodies.
2. Removal of excess wax – this is the commonest reason.

Before syringing

1. Hard wax must always be softened first to facilitate removal.
2. A doctor should always authorise ear syringing.
3. The ear should not be syringed:
   (a) if there has been recent pain accompanied by an upper respiratory tract infection;
   (b) if there is acute inflammation of the external or middle ear; or
   (c) if the tympanic membrane is perforated.
4. The meatus must always be examined with an auriscope.
5. The nurse should not undertake this procedure before having watched an experienced nurse perform it and then having performed it herself under supervision.

Equipment

Ear syringe and sterile nozzle

Auriscope
Cotton-wool buds
Cape or towel
Lotion thermometer
Kidney dish
500ml water or 1% sodium bicarbonate solution at 37°C

Method

1. Sit the patient on an upright chair with a cape or towel round his shoulders.
2. Using the auriscope, check the ear to ensure that there is no obvious inflammation or perforation of the tympanic membrane.
3. Warm the syringe by repeatedly drawing up and expelling the warm water.
4. Explain to the patient what you are going to do and how he can help by holding the receiver against his neck below his ear. A relative can help with this if the patient is unable to do so.
5. Attach the nozzle to the syringe and draw up fluid.
6. Draw the pinna upward and backward and with the same hand support the syringe nozzle when it is inserted. This protects the ear drum if the patient moves without warning.
7. Depress the syringe plunger, directing the fluid along the top and toward the back of the auditory meatus – not directly on to the tympanum.
8. Syringe until the fluid returns clear and the ear is clean on inspection with the auriscope.
9. If the wax remains hard and unmovable after three or four syringes, tell the patient to continue to use the oily drops for another four or five days and then attempt another syringing.
10. If, when the wax is removed, the ear is inflamed, refer to the doctor.
11. Dry the patient's ear with cotton-wool buds.
12. Clean and sterilise the equipment.
13. Instruct the patient to rest quietly for an hour or so as some people feel a little faint or dizzy following ear syringing.

LUNG FUNCTION TESTS

Two methods are described. The first one uses a Wright's peak flow meter and measures the peak expiratory flow rate (PEFR); the second method uses a Vitalograph dry spirometer and allows the forced vital capacity (FVC) and the forced expiratory volume in one second (FEV_1) to be measured.

Using a Wright's peak flow meter

1. Give clear instructions to the patient on how to do this test. If necessary, demonstrate yourself.
2. Allow a practice run, then take three readings and calculate the average value of these (the PEF).
3. Allow ample time for recovery between each reading.

Actual procedure

1. The patient should sit upright or stand.
2. Ask him to hold the peak flow meter in a vertical plane with the calibrated dial facing to the right. Do not allow him to cover the vent holes.
3. Ask him to take as deep a breath as possible, place his mouth over the mouthpiece, and seal his lips round it.
4. Then tell him to blow out the expired air as hard as possible in a short sharp gasp, using all his chest muscles to force it out.
5. The nurse should watch the whole procedure to ensure no leakage occurs between the mouthpiece and his lips.
6. Record the result then depress the button to release the point.
7. Rest, then try again.
8. Discard the cardboard mouthpiece after final use.

Using the Vitalograph dry spirometer

1. Prepare and explain to the patient how to do this test.
2. Fix the Vitalograph chart into the machine and set the pencil marker on the commencing mark.
3. The patient should sit upright or stand.
4. Ask him to take as deep a breath as possible, place his mouth over the disposable mouthpiece of the Vitalograph and seal his lips round it.
5. He must then exhale as hard and as quickly as possible into the Vitalograph which records the FEV_1 and FVC.
6. Two tracings should be completed.

Clinical notes

These machines may be used in general practice to assess the extent of airway obstructions on first seeing the patient. In chronic bronchitis the PEFR and FEV_1 are reduced. In a patient with suspected asthma, measurement of air flow may be used to confirm the diagnostic suspicion of the practitioner. By using these machines the progress of the disease can be followed and the effectiveness of treatment assessed.

PROCEDURES TO ASSIST RESPIRATION

Oxygen

It is usually a patient with a chronic respiratory condition who requires oxygen at home. Often an accurate percentage of oxygen is needed and this is obtained by using a Ventimask, which is available in three models allowing 24%, 28% and 35% of oxygen respectively to be delivered. Oxygen cylinders are obtainable from the chemist on an EC10, together with the head, tubing, key and mask.

Administration of oxygen

1. Assemble the equipment by attaching one end of the tubing to the outlet from the flowmeter and the other end to the mask.
2. Explain the procedure to the patient and family.
3. Wheel the equipment to the bedside.
4. Ensure the patient's airway is clear.
5. Turn on the flowmeter to the required litres per minute (normally 4–6 litres per minute).
6. Hold the mask over the patient's face initially and encourage him to relax and become used to the feel of it.
7. Position the elastic tapes of the mask comfortably, and mould the mask to fit round the face.
8. Observe the patient throughout and stay if necessary.
9. Check the oxygen supply and flow and show the patient and family how to use it.
10. Ensure that there is a second cylinder assembled with a gauge available for exchange.
11. When the oxygen therapy is discontinued, remove the mask and turn off the oxygen. Encourage the patient to drink plenty of fluids.
12. Discard the mask after final use.

Changing the cylinder

Do this away from the patient's bedside as the noise may be frightening.

1. Remove the empty cylinder from the bedside and ensure it is turned off.
2. Remove the flowmeter and gauge and place on a firm surface.
3. Remove the empty cylinder and place the full cylinder into the stand.
4. Remove the red plastic cover from the valve outlet.
5. Gently open the valve a little with the key, then close it by turning in an anti-clockwise direction. This blows out any dust before connection to the flowmeter unit.
   Caution – Do not get your face in line with the flow from the cylinder as dust may be blown into the eyes.
6. Fit the flowmeter and gauge into the new cylinder, turning it in a clockwise direction and secure firmly.
7. Gently turn on the main valve of the cylinder to register the pressure.
8. Give the relatives written instructions on how to administer oxygen and how to change the cylinder.

Precautions to be taken when using oxygen

1. Keep the cylinder away from any open fire, gas fire, electric fire, oil stove, radiator, naked light or direct sunlight.
2. Warn the patient and family not to smoke near the oxygen (within 10 feet).
3. No oil or grease should be allowed to come into contact with the oxygen fittings as this can cause an explosion.
4. Do not use any electrical apparatus such as an electric-cell bed, electric hair dryer or electric shaver. A spark from any electrical appliance may easily start a fire.
5. Avoid brisk brushing of hair, and if possible encourage the patient to wear cotton nightwear as nylon and man-made fibres encourage static electricity.
6. No metal or friction toys should be handled by the patient.
7. Spare cylinder should be stored in a cool place.
8. Always keep the cylinder turned off when not in use.
9. The room should be adequately ventilated.

Inhalations

Steam inhalations are given to soften mucus in the respiratory tract and stimulate the expectoration of secretions. They are useful to patients suffering from influenza, acute bronchitis and sinusitis. In some cases the addition of Compound Tincture of Benzoin BP (friars balsam) or menthol crystals is thought to protect the inflamed mucous membrane.

Equipment

Nelson inhaler or a 1-litre jug in a large bowl
Paper handkerchiefs
Mackintosh and towels
Kettle of hot water
Sputum mug
Inhalant, e.g. Tinct. Benz. Co BP or menthol
5ml teaspoon to measure the inhalant

Procedure

1. Fill inhaler or jug with hot water and add medicament if required (5ml to 500ml of water).
2. If a Nelson inhaler is used, cover the mouthpiece with a piece of gauze so the patient does not burn his lips, and point the spout away from the patient.
3. Assemble equipment on a suitable surface in a comfortable place for the patient.
4. Ensure the patient's bedding and furniture is protected from the hot water and inhalant with a mackintosh and towels.
5. If a jug is used place a towel over the patient's head.
6. Explain the procedure to the patient and warn him not to tilt the inhaler.
7. Supervise the inhalation for the prescribed time (usually 10 minutes).
8. Ensure careful disposal of the inhalant fluid.
9. Provide the patient with a sputum carton and tissues and encourage expectoration.
10. Tidy away the equipment, ensuring that the inhalant fluid is kept out of the reach of children.
11. Record the procedure in the nursing care plan and teach the family to repeat as required (often three times a day).
12. Always remain with children or patients who could harm themselves during this procedure.
13. Drugs may be administered in special Medihalers. These usually come complete with instructions for correct usage.

Postural drainage

The aim of postural drainage is to use gravity to assist the passage of the bronchial secretions from the periphery of the lung to the more sensitively lined bronchial tubes and thence to be expectorated. Patients with chronic lung disease such as cystic fibrosis, chronic bronchitis and bronchiectasis will have to carry out their own postural drainage at home.

Precautions

1. Do not tip cardiac and easily distressed patients unless ordered by the doctor.
2. Do not leave the patient tipped without anyone near.
3. Do not tip for longer than 20 minutes in any one position.
4. Work up to the maximum time of 20 minutes.
5. If patient shows signs of distress – sit up at once.

Procedure

1. If it is practical to tip the bed – borrow bed blocks from the Red Cross Medical Loans Depot.
2. Alternatively, for a young patient with a divan bed – instruct him to drain his lung bases by lying over the side of the bed with the forearms resting on the floor.
3. More agile patients should lie on each side in turn to drain their lung bases.
4. Another method is to tie together a bundle of magazines or newspapers, 30cm (12in) thick, and place on the bed. Put pillows on top and around and have the patient lie over them in whichever positions are necessary.
5. Babies and young children can receive postural drainage by lying over their mothers' knees.
6. The upper lobes of the lungs can be drained by positioning the patient in an upright sitting position and instructing him to lean slightly backward, or forward or sideways for short periods.
7. The physiotherapist may teach the nurses and relatives shakings and percussion movements.
8. Rolling the patient from side to side starting from the side-lying position is a useful manual aid to assist postural drainage.
9. Encourage expectoration.

For correct positioning see:
Downie, P. A. and Kennedy, P. (1981). *Lifting, Handling and Helping Patients*, pp. 81–7. Faber and Faber, London.

Tracheostomy care

A tracheostomy is an opening made into the trachea to facilitate breathing. The indications for tracheostomy are failure of respiratory function due to upper respiratory tract obstruction and conditions affecting the respiratory centre or muscles of respiration. One of the most common cases seen by the district nurse is the tracheostomy patient who has undergone a laryngectomy for carcinoma of the larynx and who is discharged home with a silver Jackson tracheostomy tube in position.

Pre-discharge arrangements

1. If possible the district nurse should visit the patient on the ward prior to his discharge to get to know both him and his family, plus the type of tracheostomy tube being used and the procedure for changing it.
2. The patient should be given a spare tracheostomy set and sterile tracheal dilators when he goes home.
3. Suction apparatus and sterile catheters should be ordered from the Health Authority Medical Loans Department.
4. Speech therapy should be organised (this is usually done by the hospital speech therapist).
5. The patient and his family should be taught how to look after the tracheostomy.

Changing an inner tube of a silver tracheostomy tube

Equipment

Basic dressing pack and extra gauze swabs
Forceps
Johnson and Johnson keyhole dressing (if available)
Tracheal dilators
Duplicate tracheostomy set
Electric suction apparatus and sterile catheters (adult 14–18 FG, child 5–13 FG)
5% sodium bicarbonate solution
Skin cleansing lotion such as Normasol sachets
2 receivers
Disposable gloves
Medical wipes
Scissors
Receiver containing wire brush

Method

1. The procedure is explained to the patient and the equipment assembled on a clean table at the patient's side. A writing pad and pencil should be kept near the patient to aid communication.
2. He should be sitting upright in a comfortable position with his head slightly tilted back.
3. Check that the tapes on the outer tube are clean and secure and that the suction apparatus is working.
4. Wash your hands and open out the packs and the equipment, pour the Normasol into the galipot.
5. Perform tracheal suction if this is necessary.
6. Put on disposable gloves, put towel round the patient and remove the inner tube into the receiver.
7. Clean this tube (the inner tube) thoroughly using the 5% sodium bicarbonate solution and wire brush. Rinse under cold running water then place in sterilising solution for three minutes.
8. Discard gloves. Wash hands, then either put on a clean pair of sterile gloves or use forceps to clean around the patient's outer tracheostomy tube using swabs and Normasol.
9. Dry the sterile inner tube with a sterile towel or gauze. Check that the outer tube is clear.
10. Insert the inner tube and, if a Jackson tube is used, check that the clip is in the correct position to secure the tube.
11. Check that the tapes are secure.
12. Remove the towel and make the patient comfortable and ensure that a call bell and pad and pencil are within easy reach.
13. Clear away the equipment. Clean and sterilise the instruments and brush.
14. Record the procedure in the nursing care plan.

It is a good idea for the patient's spouse to stay and observe the procedure and give moral support. A tracheostomy can be very frightening at first to both the patient and his family and the nurse must be aware of this and be prepared to offer much advice and support.

Changing the outer silver tracheostomy tube

Equipment

Same as for changing the inner tube – no need for a wire brush and receiver as a new tube is to be inserted.

Pair of sterile gloves
Sterile tracheostomy tube set of the correct size
Receiver with 5% sodium bicarbonate solution

Method

1. The equipment is assembled as before and the patient positioned in the same way.
2. Suction apparatus is checked to be certain that it is in working order.
3. Wash the hands and open the dressing pack and new tracheostomy set. Pour the lotion into the galipot.
4. Check that the tapes of the new tracheostomy tube are secure and of adequate length.
5. Carry out tracheal suction if needed.
6. Arrange the towel round the patient, then using forceps clean the area around the tracheostomy tube with gauze moistened with Normasol.
7. Put on the sterile gloves.
8. Cut the tapes holding the tube in position with the scissors and remove the soiled tube, placing it into a receiver of 5% sodium bicarbonate solution.
9. Immediately, during inspiration, insert the new tube and remove the introducer. Obviously it is easier if there are two people to carry out this procedure – one to remove the old tube and one to insert the new sterile one. In some cases a sterile water-soluble lubricant may need to be applied on gauze to the new tube.
10. The inner tube is then inserted. Check that the clip is in the correct position to secure the tube.
11. Tie the tapes securely and comfortably.
12. Clean the area around the tube with a moistened swab and dry well.
13. Remove the towel and clear away the equipment.
14. Make the patient comfortable as before and make sure that he is breathing satisfactorily.
15. Record the procedure in the nursing care plan and report on the condition of the stoma.

16. Clean the dirty tubes and introducer and send them for sterilisation. Ensure a duplicate set is available.

BLADDER PROCEDURES

Catheterisation

Whenever catheterisation is carried out it must be a sterile procedure and an aseptic technique should be used to avoid introducing bacteria into the bladder.

Pre-packed sterile equipment is best but where none is available, items which should be sterile can be boiled in water or sterilised in an approved solution. Catheters are obtained either through the district health authority or from the chemist on prescription. Some areas have a CSSD for the use of district nurses but in other parts of the country dressing packs must also be obtained on prescription.

It is important that the nurse should explain the procedure in terms understood and accepted by the patient before commencing.

Equipment

Large dressing pack or catheterisation pack
Large sterile receiver
Small sterile receiver for lotion (for example – Salvodil)
Measuring jug
2 sterile catheters 16–24 FG of the appropriate make
Sterile gloves
Paper bags for soiled swabs
Specimen jar if required
20ml syringe ⎫
Sterile water ⎬ If catheter is to remain in situ
Uribag or spigot ⎬
Uribag holder ⎭
Incopad to protect the bed

Procedure

1. Protect the bed with an Incopad and make the patient comfortable in a dorsal position.
2. Prepare a clean working surface and assemble all the equipment needed, including containers for the disposal of soiled equipment, linen and dressings.
3. Ensure there is adequate lighting.

4. Wash the hands thoroughly and dry on a sterile towel from the pack.
5. Ask the patient to draw up her feet and then let her knees fall apart. If the patient is unable to co-operate and help, the nurse may need to ask a relative to help support the patient's legs.
6. Put on sterile gloves (or use sterile forceps).
7. Place a sterile towel over the abdomen and one on the bed between the legs.
8. Carry out vulval swabbing with the warm sterile solution.
9. Place a large receiver on the towel between the legs.
10. Cut off the end of the outer plastic bag round the catheter and withdraw the inner bag.
11. Open the inner bag without touching the catheter and, holding the catheter, still in the plastic bag, with one hand, separate the labia with the other.
12. Insert the tip of the catheter into the urethra and pass it for about 10cm, withdrawing the plastic bag at the same time. A specimen, if required, may be collected in this inner bag at this point.
13. Allow the rest of the urine to drain from the catheter into the large receiver. If retention is the problem 200ml is released at 30-minute intervals.
14. Check the size of the balloon before injecting the correct amount of sterile water into the balloon of the self-retaining catheter.
15. Affix drainage as necessary, or insert a spigot.
16. Make the patient comfortable, then clear up the equipment.
17. Measure the urine in the receiver. Note any significant observations and record the findings on the nursing treatment card.
18. Before leaving ensure that the catheter and drainage are satisfactory.
19. Make sure that the patient and relatives have understood your instructions about catheter care and toilet.

Some district nurses prefer to use forceps to achieve a non-touch technique; others wear sterile gloves. Whichever method used does not matter, so long as it is a sterile procedure.

Advice
The following advice should be given to patients (and their

relatives) with indwelling catheters and continuous bladder drainage.

1. Drink at least one litre of fluid a day.
2. Do not lift the bag above bladder level so that there is no back flow of urine into the bladder.
3. Empty the bag at least every eight hours and pay strict attention to handwashing before and after the procedure.
4. Report to your nurse or GP:
    (a) urine with a foul odour, cloudiness or bloodstaining
    (b) a rise in temperature for a day or two
    (c) urethral discharge
    (d) abdominal pain
    (e) reduction in the amount of urine passed, accompanied by abdominal distension and pain.
5. Wash the urethral meatal area daily with soap and water and dry well. Some doctors prescribe an antiseptic cream such as chlorhexidine to apply around this area.
6. Save a specimen of urine for the nurse or doctor to test if you have any of the symptoms mentioned above (4).
7. Keep a record of the measurement of the amount of urine passed in 24 hours if you think that it is less than normal. Also record intake.
8. Because of the danger of introducing an infection into the bladder, the drainage system should be kept closed. If four-hourly release of urine is ordered by the doctor, a gate clip should be used rather than a spigot.
9. Report to the nurse or GP any skin rashes on the legs which may occur if a leg bag with rubber straps is worn.

Bladder irrigation

The type of bladder irrigation performed in the home is usually intermittent in nature, and is carried out using a 50ml bladder syringe. Because there is a high risk of introducing infection using this method of irrigation it is essential for it to be carried out as a sterile procedure.

Equipment

    1 sterile 50ml bladder syringe
    2 pairs sterile gloves
    Bag for rubbish

2 sterile measuring jugs
Sterile receiver
New drainage bag
Irrigation fluid, for example, sterile normal saline
Container of hot water to warm the fluid
Incopad or towel to protect the bed

Procedure

1. Assemble the equipment.
2. Explain the procedure to the patient.
3. Make him comfortable in a semi-recumbent position with his buttocks on the Incopad, and clothing removed from below the waist.
4. Wash your hands, put on gloves and place the sterile receiver between the patient's legs.
5. Remove the old drainage bag and allow the catheter to drain into the receiver while the old drainage bag is emptied and dispensed with.
6. Change to a new pair of sterile gloves and aspirate the catheter prior to irrigation.
7. Use warm normal saline (or other solution prescribed by the doctor) to wash out the bladder.
8. Care should be taken to ensure that the same amount of fluid which is injected is being aspirated.
9. Reconnect the new drainage bag.
10. Observe the aspirate and record any findings on the treatment card.
11. Clear away the equipment and sterilise non-disposable items.
12. Ensure that the catheter is draining and that the patient and carers understand the care of the catheter.

GYNAECOLOGICAL PROCEDURES

Vaginal examinations

High vaginal swabs are taken to test for the presence of micro-organisms so that the correct treatment is prescribed.

Equipment

Disposable gloves
Towel to protect the bed
Sterile swabs

Sanipad (if needed)
Warm antiseptic solution
Bag for refuse
1 charcoal swab
2 plain swabs
Bottle of Stuart's medium
Bottle of trichomonas medium
Pathology forms signed by the doctor
Adequate lighting

Procedure

1. Explain to the patient what you want to do, what is entailed, and why it is necessary.
2. If the patient is mobile, ask her to go to the toilet to empty her bladder, or offer her a bedpan.
3. Prepare the working surface, lay out the equipment and protect the bed.
4. Position the patient in either a left lateral or dorsal position and ensure that she is warm and comfortable.
5. Wash your hands and put on the gloves.
6. Proceed with vulval toilet.
7. Separate the labia and insert the speculum with the blades closed and the greatest diameter in the antero-posterior plane. DO NOT USE A LUBRICANT.
8. If resistance is met, ask the patient to bear down or cough.
9. Rotate the speculum through 90° and open up the blades to reveal the cervix.
10. Swab the fornices with the 3 swabs and return them temporarily to their containers while you close, rotate and remove the speculum.
11. Break off 2 swabs into the trichomonas medium and the charcoal swab into the Stuart's medium.
12. Make the patient comfortable – apply a sanipad if necessary.
13. Clear away the equipment – wash and sterilise the speculum.
14. Label the swabs clearly and complete the request form. Store in a refrigerator until they can be sent to the laboratory.
15. Record the procedure and any findings in the nursing records and report to the GP as necessary.

Vaginal douche

This procedure is carried out if the patient has an unpleasant

vaginal discharge. It may also be used following radiotherapy to the
cervix to clear away the debris. As always – careful explanation and
reassurance are essential.

Equipment
    Disposable sterile gloves
    Sterile swabs
    Warm douche solution in a sterile jug (40°C)
    Bag for refuse
    Bedpan
    Waterproof protection for the bed
    Sanipad
    Sterile douche can
    Rubber tubing
    Gate clip
    Douche nozzle

Procedure
1. Ensure that the patient empties her bladder before the
   procedure begins.
2. Protect the bed and assemble all the equipment including
   containers for the disposal of soiled equipment, linen and
   dressings.
3. Prepacked sterile equipment is best but, where none is
   available, the items which should be sterile can be boiled in
   water for 10 minutes or sterilised in an approved solution.
4. Ensure that the patient is warm and in a comfortable
   semi-recumbent dorsal position on a bedpan.
5. Wash your hands and put on the sterile gloves.
6. Carry out vulval swabbing with the warm sterile solution.
7. Place the douche can on a table near the patient at a level of
   about 12 inches above the mattress.
8. Inspect the douche nozzle to ensure it is not damaged and
   release the gate clip slightly from the rubber tubing (while
   holding the nozzle over the bedpan) to expel air – then
   re-clamp the gate clip.
9. Separate the labia with the left hand and gently insert the
   douche nozzle for about 3½ inches into the vagina in an
   upward and backward direction.
10. Release the gate clip with the left hand.
11. Slowly turn the nozzle from side to side as the fluid is released.

12. When the douche is completed, remove the nozzle and place it in the douche can.
13. Before removing the bedpan from the patient, make sure the vagina is emptied – to do this sit the patient forward and ask her to cough.
14. Leave the patient dry and comfortable with a sanipad in position.
15. Clear away, and sterilise the equipment.
16. Inspect the amount of debris and type of fluid returned and record the significant observations on the nursing treatment card and report to the GP if necessary.

Cervical cytology

This is a diagnostic procedure, usually carried out in the health centre, in family planning clinics or well-women clinics or by the GP. Scrapings are taken from the neck of the cervix, deposited on a glass slide, fixed with pure alcohol and sent to the laboratory for cytological examination. Some district nurses participate in well-women clinics and may be required to carry out this procedure.

Equipment

Cusco's speculum
Tissues
Ayre's spatula
Disposable gloves
Fixative
2 microscope slides with the ground end labelled in pencil with the patient's full name and the date
Cytology request form
Claim form FP74
Light – Angle-poise
Plastic transport container

Procedure

1. Explain to the patient what is to be done and ask if she wishes to go to the toilet before you start.
2. Ask her to strip from the waist downward.
3. Position the patient on the couch according to your preference – either in the left lateral or dorsal position.
4. Ensure the equipment is at hand and in working order.

5. Use warm water to lubricate the speculum as it is less of a shock to the patient if the speculum is warm, and the use of jelly spoils the smear. Put on gloves.
6. Separate the labia and position the Angle-poise lamp.
7. Insert the speculum with the blades closed, with the greatest diameter in the antero-posterior plane.
8. Rotate and open the blades to show the cervix.
9. Apply the Ayre's spatula to the cervix and rotate it using gentle pressure so as to obtain a scraping of the mucus containing the desquamated cells.
10. Close, rotate and remove the speculum.
11. Prepare the microscope slides, using gentle even sweeps. Do not go over the same area twice.
12. Apply the fixative immediately and allow the slides to dry before placing them in the plastic transport box.
13. Make sure the slides are both labelled with the patient's name and the date.
14. Ask the patient to dress.
15. Complete the request form with the following information:
    Full name, address and date of birth
    NHS number and name and address of GP
    Marital status and parity of the patient
    Type of contraception used (if any)
    Date of the first day of the last menstrual period
    Date of the last smear (if known)
    Any grounds for clinical suspicion.
16. Complete the claim form FP 74 if both of the following conditions apply:
    (a) The patient has not had a smear taken during the last 5 years (unless this is a repeat smear being taken at the request of the laboratory).
    (b) The patient is 35 years old or over or has had three or more children.
17. Ask the patient to sign the claim form and explain about the notification of results of the smear test.
18. Clear away the equipment and clean and sterilise the speculum.

Clinical notes

Carcinoma of the cervix is the second commonest form of cancer found in women. It can occur at any age but is most common in the

40 to 50 year age-group, and in women who have had a large family early in their lives. It is rare in unmarried women who are virgins and therefore it would appear to be linked in some way with sexual intercourse.

Routine cervical cytology has been of great value in detecting the pre-clinical symptomless state known as 'carcinoma-in-situ'. A positive smear is usually followed by a cone biopsy from the cervix. In young women wishing to have children this may be all that is necessary to remove the whole area of malignant cells. Regular smears are of vital importance because malignant changes in the cells of the cervix can spread locally very quickly. The treatment of choice is surgery followed by radiotherapy and in the early stages of the disease the prognosis following therapy is good.

Vaginal pessary

There are two types of vaginal pessary which the district nurse may encounter in the course of her work.

Medicated pessaries (which are inserted by the patient herself) are used to treat vaginal infections such as *Candida albicans* (thrush). They are best inserted at night when the patient is lying in a dorsal position as they do melt and drain out of the vagina when the patient is up and about. This means that she has to wear a pad to protect her clothing. The nurse must emphasise the need to complete the course of treatment and not to stop as the symptoms subside.

The other type of pessary is a device for supporting a displaced uterus by insertion into the vagina.

Indications for pessary treatment
1. The patient prefers pessary treatment to the alternative of pelvic surgery.
2. The prolapse is amenable to pessary support.
3. The patient is not fit for surgery.
4. The patient wishes to delay surgery temporarily (for example another pregnancy is anticipated).

Disadvantages
1. In the past the old rubber ring pessaries got a bad reputation because they caused a profuse purulent discharge.
2. Pessaries needed changing every four to six months.

3. If ill fitting, pessaries can cause discomfort, constipation, dyspareunia and dysuria.
4. If too tight or left in too long, vaginal ulceration will occur.

It is very important that an experienced doctor should fit the initial pessary to ensure that no complications, due to ill-fitting, occur. The district nurse will then be asked to change the pessary at prescribed intervals.

Types of pessary

Ring pessaries are used to treat prolapses.

Semi-soft vinyl ring pessaries are useful when there is senile shrinkage of the introitus which makes insertion of a big enough ring difficult. They are easy to remove.

Semi-rigid polythene ring pessaries are best. They are easy to insert but may be difficult to extract.

Rigid bakelite pessaries with bars may be used to prevent a large prolapse from herniating through the ring. By this stage, however, the pelvic floor is usually too stretched to retain it, and so the district nurse rarely sees this type of pessary.

The Hodge pessary is used to correct retroversion of the uterus. It is a rigid pessary of bakelite or Perspex, oblong in shape and having an 'S' curve. It helps to maintain the anteverted position by pressing on the utero-sacral ligaments. It is only left in position for a few weeks and is initially fitted by a gynaecologist.

Equipment for changing a pessary

   Towel to protect the bed
   New pessary of the correct size and material
   Container for the old pessary
   2 pairs of sterile gloves
   Lubricant
   Cotton-wool swabs
   Warm antiseptic solution
   Good light

Procedure

1. While the patient goes to the toilet, prepare the working surface, lay out equipment and protect the bed.
2. Ensure the patient understands the procedure and is warm and comfortable.

3. Put the patient in the left lateral position.
4. Wash your hands and put on disposable gloves.
5. Lubricate the exterior of the vagina/vulva.
6. Insert the index finger and remove the old pessary.
7. Carry out vulval toilet if there is much discharge. Change gloves.
8. Compress the new pessary into a long ovoid shape and gently push it into the vagina (after lubrication) where it resumes its circular shape, and takes up a position in the coronal plane.
9. Dry the vulva.
10. Ask the patient to stand up and bend over to ensure that the pessary is fitting properly and is comfortable.
11. Clear away the equipment and dispose of the old pessary.

VENEPUNCTURE

There are always technicians or doctors in hospital who are prepared to take specimens of blood from patients. In the community, however, it is often the district nursing sister who is required to carry out this procedure. Policies vary in different parts of the country but the nurse should receive instructions in venepuncture if she is to carry out this procedure as a routine part of her work.

Equipment needed

Hypodermic syringe of the appropriate size – depending on the amount of blood required
Needle size 21 s.w.g.
Steret or spirit swabs
Medical wipe
Container for blood
Pathological request forms
Venous tourniquet or sphygmomanometer

Procedure

1. Position the patient comfortably with his sleeve rolled up and the arm supported on a table or pillow.
2. Protect the table or bedclothes with a towel or mackintosh.
3. Wash your hands and assemble the equipment.
4. Apply tourniquet or sphygmomanometer cuff inflated to 80mm Hg so as to occlude the venous return.

5. Loosen the bottle tops because no delay must occur once blood has been taken. If a Sequestrene sample is required the specimen bottles must not be left with their tops off.
6. Check again the signed blood request forms to ensure the correct bottles and amounts of blood are collected.
7. Examine the patient's arm and choose the appropriate vein to be used.
8. Swab the skin with a medi-swab and allow to dry as un-evaporated spirit stings when the needle is inserted.
9. Check the syringe and needle to ensure it is patent and the plunger moves freely.
10. Insert the needle in the direction of the flow of blood.
11. Draw up the required amount of blood.
12. Release the tourniquet/cuff.
13. Withdraw the needle and cover the point of insertion with a tissue.
14. Ask the patient or a relative to press the tissue gently over the area to stop bleeding. Alternatively, the elbow can be flexed.
15. Quickly remove the needle and fill the appropriate bottles with the correct amount of blood, being careful not to spill any.
16. Gently mix the Sequestrene sample.
17. Break the needle and syringe hilt to prevent any further misuse and dispose of these safely according to district policy.
18. Check that haemostasis has been achieved and apply a patch dressing.
19. Complete the request forms and label the samples with the full name, age, sex, time and date.
20. Wash your hands and pack up the nursing bag.
21. Ensure the patient is comfortable.
22. Record in the patient's medical (and nursing) notes that a blood sample has been taken.

Special notes

1. Blood from jaundiced patients and from those with suspected hepatitis should be sent to the pathological laboratory sealed in a polythene bag and labelled 'hepatitis risk'. The request form should be marked with a yellow diagonal line.
2. Wear gloves if possible when carrying out venepuncture on this type of patient to prevent skin contact with the blood.

3. If possible take blood for serum calcium investigations without using a cuff or tourniquet.
4. In all cases, venous return should be obstructed for as short a time as possible.

There should be a laboratory chart kept in the health centre treatment room to indicate the volume of blood required for haematological investigations and the colour code on the bottle labels.

FINANCIAL BENEFITS
AND HELP

Many elderly, sick and disabled people are unaware of the financial aid to which they are entitled because of their condition. The district nurse should be able to advise her patients as to their possible entitlements and suggest that they obtain the relevant leaflets from the local Social Security Department, the Post Office, Citizens Advice Bureaux or, in some cases, the public library or health centre. Leaflet numbers and actual financial payments are not included here as they are constantly changing.

CONTRIBUTORY BENEFITS

Maternity benefits
Sickness benefits
Invalidity benefit – replaces sickness benefit after 28 weeks of illness
Unemployment benefit – if unemployed and capable of work
Earnings-related supplement – paid after the first 12 days of an interruption of employment and lasts a maximum of six months
Widow's benefits
Retirement pension
Death grant – amount varies according to the age of the deceased

NON-CONTRIBUTORY BENEFITS

Child benefit
Family Income Supplement – earnings related
Supplementary Benefits – pension or allowance
Attendance Allowance – may be claimed by a relative on behalf of an elderly or disabled person who, because of severe physical or mental disabilities, needs frequent attention

throughout the day (and often during the night). The requirement must be of six months' duration before a claim can be submitted

Mobility Allowance – paid to people from the age of five to pensionable age who are severely disabled and unable to walk, or have great difficulty in walking

Severe Disablement Allowance (SDA)

Invalid Care Allowance – paid to working men and women who have to stay at home to care for a disabled relative receiving the Attendance Allowance

Industrial Injuries Benefit

BIBLIOGRAPHY

The following titles provide a wealth of information concerning benefits and entitlements. They are regularly updated.

Disability Rights Handbook (Annual). Available from the Disability Alliance Educational and Research Association, 25 Denmark Street, London WC2H 8NJ.

Guide to the Social Services edited by B. Preston, published by the Family Welfare Association, 501–505 Kingsland Road, London E8 4AU.

Non-Contributory Benefits for Disabled People Handbook published by HMSO, London.

Social Services Year Book published by Longman Group Limited, 6th Floor, Westgate House, The High, Harlow CM20 1NE.

Further Reading

In addition to the books and papers mentioned in the references and bibliography at the end of some of the chapters, the following is a select list of titles which will be found useful by district nurses.

Anderson, D. J. (1981). *Drugs and the Community Nurse*, Royal College of Nursing, London.

Baly, M. (ed) (1981). *A New Approach to District Nursing.* William Heinemann Medical Books Limited, London.

Berber, J. H. and Kratz, C. R. (jt eds) (1980). *Towards Team Care.* Churchill Livingstone, Edinburgh.

Chapman, C. M. (1982). *Sociology for Nurses*, 2nd edition. Baillière Tindall, Eastbourne.

Equipment for the Disabled. A series of books published by the Oxford Area Health Authority on behalf of the DHSS. Available from Equipment for the Disabled, 2 Foredown Drive, Portslade, Brighton BN4 2BB.

Gaffin, J. (1981). *The Nurse and the Welfare State.* H. M. + M. Publishers (John Wiley and Sons Limited, Chichester).

Hicks, D. (1976). *Primary Health Care.* HMSO, London.

Kark, S. L. (1981). *The Practice of Community-Oriented Primary Health Care.* Appleton Century Crofts, East Horwalk, CT.

Skeet, M. H. and Crout, E. (1977). *Health Needs Help.* Blackwell Scientific Publications Limited, Oxford.

Thomas, D. (1982). *The Experience of Handicap.* Methuen and Co Limited, London.

Tschudin, V. (1982). *Counselling Skills for Nurses*, Baillière Tindall, Eastbourne.

White, R. (1978). *Social Change and the Development of the Nursing Profession: Study of the Poor Law Nursing Service, 1848–1948.* Kimpton Medical Publications, London.

Useful Organisations

This is only a random selection of the many organisations which may be able to offer help, advice and guidance both to patients, district nurses or others working in the community. The local Citizens Advice Bureaux will have lists of local organisations.

For more extensive information the following books are recommended:
Directory for the Disabled, edited by A. Darnbrough and D. Kinrade and published by Woodhead-Faulkner, Cambridge CB2 3PF. It is regularly updated.
Help Starts Here. This is specifically related to children. It can be obtained from the Voluntary Council for Handicapped Children, National Children's Bureau, 8 Wakley Street, London EC1V 7QE.

Action on Smoking and Health (ASH) 5–11 Mortimer Street, London W1N 7RH	01-637 9843
Age Concern England (National Old People's Welfare Council) Bernard Sunley House, 60 Pitcairn Road Mitcham, Surrey CR4 3LL	01-640 5431
Alcoholics Anonymous PO Box 514, 11 Redcliffe Gardens London SW10 9BQ	01-352 5493/9779
Association to Aid Sexual and Personal Relationships of Disabled People (SPOD) 286 Camden Road, London N7 0BJ	01-607 8851
Association for Disabled Professionals (ADP) The Stables, 73 Pound Road Banstead, Surrey SM7 2HU	(Burgh Heath) 07373 52366
British Association of the Hard of Hearing 7–11 Armstrong Road, London W3 7JL	01-743 1110

British Diabetic Association
10 Queen Anne Street, London W1M 0BD　　　　　01-323 1531

British Epilepsy Association
Crowthorne House, New Wokingham Road
Wokingham, Berkshire RG11 3AY　　　(Crowthorne) 0344 773122

British Gas Home Service Department
326 High Holborn, London WC1V 7PT　　　　　01-242 0789

British Red Cross Society
9 Grosvenor Crescent, London SW1X 7EJ　　　　01-235 5454

British Rheumatism and Arthritis Association
6 Grosvenor Crescent, London SW1X 7ER　　　　01-235 0902

British Wireless for the Blind Fund
224 Great Portland Street, London W1N 6AA　　　01-388 1266

Cancer After-Care and Rehabilitation Society (CARE)
Lodge Cottage, Church Lane
Timsbury, Bath BA3 1LF　　　　　　　　　　076170731

Chest, Heart and Stroke Association
Tavistock House North
Tavistock Square, London WC1H 9JE　　　　　01-387 3012

Colostomy Welfare Group
38–9 Eccleston Square, London SW1V 1PB　　　01-828 5175

CRACK (The Young Arm of the Multiple Sclerosis Society)
286 Munster Road, Fulham, London SW6 6AP　　01-381 4022

Crossroads Care Attendant Schemes Ltd
94a Coton Road, Rugby
Warwickshire CV21 4LN　　　　　　　　　078873653

CRUSE
Cruse House, 126 Sheen Road
Richmond, Surrey TW9 1UR　　　　　　　　01-940 4818

Depressives Associated
19 Merley Ways, Wimborne Minster
Dorset BH21 1QN　　　　　　　　　　　0202 883957

Disabled Living Foundation (DLF)
380–384 Harrow Road, London W9 2HU   01-289 6111

Disablement Income Group Advisory Service (DIG)
Attlee House, 28 Commercial Street
London E1 6LR   01-247 2128

Down's Children's Association
4 Oxford Street, London W1R 1PA   01-580 0511

Elderly Invalids Fund
131 Middlesex Street, London E1 7JF   01-621 1624

Electricity Council
Marketing Department (Publications Section)
30 Millbank, London SW1P 4RD   01-834 2333

Family Planning Association
27 Mortimer Street, London W1N 7RJ   01-636 7866

Federation of Alcoholic Rehabilitation Establishments
  (FARE)
3 Grosvenor Crescent, London SW1X 7EE   01-235 0609

GRACE (Mrs Gould's Residential Advisory Centre for
  the Elderly)
PO Box 71, Cobham, Surrey KT11 2JR   09326 2928/5765

Health Education Council
78 New Oxford Street, London WC1A 1AH   01-637 1881

Help the Aged
1 St James's Walk, London EC1R 0BE   01-253 0253

Ileostomy Association of Great Britain and Ireland
Central Office, Amblehurst House
Chobham, Woking, Surrey GU24 8PZ   (Chobham) 09905 8277

Information Service for the Disabled
see Disabled Living Foundation

In Touch
BBC Publications
PO Box 234, London SE1 3TH   01-407 6961

Invalids at Home Trust 23 Farm Avenue, London NW2 2BJ (money for equipment)	01-452 2074
The Leonard Cheshire Foundation 26–9 Maunsel Street, London SW1P 2QN	01-828 1822
The Marie Curie Memorial Foundation 28 Belgrave Square, London SW1X 8QG (for night nursing service)	01-235 3325
Mastectomy Association 26 Harrison Street, London WC1H 8JG	01-837 0908
The Medic-Alert Foundation 11–13 Clifton Terrace, London N4 3JP	01-263 8596
Mental After-Care Association Eagle House, 110 Jermyn Street London SW1Y 6HB	01-839 5953
The Mental Health Foundation 8 Hallam Street, London W1N 6BH	01-580 0145
Migraine Trust 45 Great Ormond Street, London WC1N 3HD	01-278 2676
MIND (The National Association for Mental Health) 22 Harley Street, London W1N 2ED	01-637 0741
Multiple Sclerosis Society of Great Britain and Northern Ireland 25 Effie Road, London SW6 1EE	01-381 4022
Action for Research into Multiple Sclerosis (ARMS) 11 Dartmouth Street, London SW1H 9BL	01-222 3224
Muscular Dystrophy Group of Great Britain and Northern Ireland Nattrass House, 35 Macaulay Road London SW5 0QP	01-720 8055
National Council for Carers and their Elderly Dependants 29 Chilworth Mews, London W2 3RG	01-262 1451

National Schizophrenia Fellowship
78–9 Victoria Road, Surbiton
Surrey KT6 4JT   01-390 3651/2

National Society for Cancer Relief
Michael Sobell House, 30 Dorset Square
London NW1 6QL   01-402 8125

The Open Door Association (Agoraphobia)
c/o 447 Pensby Road
Heswall, Wirral
Merseyside L61 9PQ

Parkinson's Disease Society
36 Portland Place, London W1N 3DG   01-323 1174

Partially Sighted Society
40 Wordsworth Street, Hove
East Sussex BN3 5BH   (Brighton) 0273 736053

Pensioners Link Limited (formerly Task Force)
17 Balfe Street, London N1 9EB   01-278 5501

The Phobics Society
c/o 4 Cheltenham Road
Chorlton-cum-Hardy
Manchester M21 1AN

Royal Association for Disability and Rehabilitation
    (RADAR)
25 Mortimer Street, London W1N 8AB   01-637 5400

Royal National Institute for the Blind (RNIB)
224 Great Portland Street, London W1N 6AA   01-388 1266

Royal National Institute for the Deaf (RNID)
105 Gower Street, London WC1E 6AH   01-387 8033

Royal Society for Mentally Handicapped Children and Adults
    (MENCAP)
123 Golden Lane, London EC1Y 0RT   01-253 9433

Spastics Society
12 Park Crescent, London W1N 4EQ   01-636 5020

Spinal Injuries Association (SIA)
Yeoman House, St James' Lane,
London N10 3DF   01-444 2121

Telephones for the Blind Fund
Mynthurst, Leigh
Reigate, Surrey RH2 7BB   02938 62546

Urinary Conduit Association
8 Coniston Close, Dane Bank
Denton, Manchester M34 2EW   061-336 8818

Women's National Cancer Control Campaign
1 South Audley Street, London W1Y 5DQ   01-499 7532

Index